OVERCOMING
CANCER

OVERCOMING CANCER

The 5 Most Powerful Tools for Fighting Cancer

GARY NULL, PhD

Gary Null Publishing

Library of Congress Cataloging-in-Publication Data is available on file.

Cover design by Jane Sheppard
Cover photograph by iStockphoto

Print ISBN: 978-1-5107-1570-7
Ebook ISBN: 978-1-5107-1571-4

Printed in the United States of America

Table of Contents

Introduction

One word strikes more fear into a person's mind than any other: cancer. The disease has evolved into a national crisis that touches each and every one of us. The immense physical, mental, emotional, and financial toll that comes with a cancer diagnosis affects patients, their families, and entire communities. In 2017, approximately 600,000 Americans will lose their lives to cancer, and the forecast shows no signs of improving.[1] Latest estimates tell us that 41 percent of all Americans will be diagnosed with cancer during their lifetimes and 21 percent of the population will lose their lives to this devastating disease.[2] The majority of individuals who fight the battle against cancer are treated with the standard orthodox therapy, or the "official treatment." Rarely do they question their oncologists; rather they believe they are in the best possible hands with their physicians' advanced education, their knowledge of the most effective treatments, and their access to the latest modern research.

Patients assume these therapies have been proven safe and effective through rigorous clinical testing. They feel assured that any treatments available to improve the chance of survival will be found in the "official" medical journals and sanctioned by leading cancer institutions such as Memorial Sloan-Kettering

Cancer Center and the Mayo Clinic. If a promising new cancer treatment comes along, we trust that it will be supported and funded by organizations such as the National Cancer Institute and the American Cancer Society. When new articles announce that a silver-bullet cancer therapy is just around the corner, and encourage us to fund these institutions, we believe that our contributions will be applied with the best of intentions for the public good in the war against cancer. Unfortunately, these institutions and their motivations do not hold up under close scrutiny. Instead, our belief in and support of the cancer industry and the medical-industrial complex promotes a corrupt system defined by endless greed, bad science, and appalling disregard for human life.

The most important progress in preventing and treating cancer has not come from official institutions but from those who are regarded as renegades and espouse alternative medicine. Despite the well-documented success independent researchers have had using alternative therapies, they are rejected by mainstream medicine. Scientists and physicians who provide evidence of a cancer cure that diverts from surgery, chemotherapy, or radiation are likely to be vilified, silenced, or drummed out of the medical profession in the United States altogether. Consequently, very little progress has been made. We have been waging an official war on cancer for more than forty-five years. Hundreds of billions of dollars have been spent to fund legions of scientists, physicians, nurses, and public health officials in a campaign to end this devastating affliction; yet the survival rates for most cancers—including our number-one killer, lung cancer—remain dismally low.

In this book we'll look at the shortcomings of the standard approach to prevention and treatment of cancer and the promise of alternative approaches. In the introduction I'll summarize why so little progress has been made, how the cancer establishment has a stake in suppressing information about alternative treatments, and why standard approaches are inadequate. Then, in the bulk of the book, I'll provide the latest research about foods and supplements that boost the body's immune system in order to prevent and reverse cancer. I'll explore several successful alternative cancer therapies now practiced today in clinics across the globe—therapies whose safety and efficacy are supported by reliable peer-reviewed scientific findings. During the past thirty-five years, I have spent a great deal of time studying these treatments while visiting clinics around the world and interviewing thousands of patients. I'll discuss those treatments that have the highest rate of success and present testimonials by patients who, despite being told by conventional doctors that they would not survive, ultimately triumphed against cancer using alternative medicine. This is not to suggest that other holistic cancer treatments not included are unsuccessful. However, I have been unable to verify their effectiveness.

I have also included dozens of delicious and healthy recipes to strengthen and support the immune system in its fight against cancer.

What Is Cancer?

Cancer is a group of diseases in which abnormal cells, instead of being killed by the body's immune system, multiply and spread. The cells no longer follow the rules for the usual orderly progression of growth and become renegades. Cancer can attack any part of the body and may spread to other parts. The sites most often affected are the skin, the digestive organs, the lungs, the prostate gland, and the female breasts.

A healthy cell starts out as immature and then goes through routine changes to mature. As a mature cell, it performs whatever job in the body it is supposed to do, and then it gets old and dies. Along the way, the active mature cell needs maintenance. There are genes in the cell that do the job of repairing mistakes and keeping the cell in running order.

Cancer occurs when the cell doesn't mature, doesn't repair its mistakes, or doesn't die. There are two types of cancer: those that form tumors and those that don't. When these outlaw cancer cells are regular building-block cells, like cells in the breast, lung, prostate, or skin, tumors occur. These cancers show up as abnormal masses or tumors because the cells are replicating out of control, heaping up into big masses, and killing the normal cells around them.

Cancers can also be in non–building-block cells. This type of cancer doesn't produce a tumor and occurs in the cells of the blood. The blood cells go out of control, resulting in cancers like leukemia and lymphomas. These blood cells remain immature. They proliferate and push out and kill the regular healthy mature blood cells. They show up in the bone marrow or clog up the lymph nodes or the spleen.

Then there is a really tricky part of cancer, and the part that can lead to death, which is when the aberrant cells migrate. They metastasize and invade other parts of the body, setting up shop in parts of the body distant from their original site. For instance, prostate cancer likes to invade the bones and brain. Breast cancer cells like the bones and the liver. The cancer cells develop the ability to spread by making special enzymes that cut through cell walls and travel through the blood.

What makes the cell go haywire? No one can answer for sure. But what can we do to prevent cancer? What can we do to fight cancer once the cells have gone out of control? There is a lot to say in response to these questions. First, poisonous elements from the environment can cause the cell to become cancerous, things like asbestos and cigarettes. But it also turns out that some people are more inclined to get cancer than others are. Genetic predisposition and environmental assaults appear to provide the powerful one-two punch.

The Cancer Establishment's Failed War

In December 1971, with much fanfare, President Richard Nixon declared war on cancer. Forty-five years later, America is realizing it has been fighting a losing battle. The American Cancer Society reports the following:

- Approximately 600,000 Americans will die from cancer over the next twelve months (1,500 deaths each day).
- Nearly 1.7 million individuals will be diagnosed with cancer this year, as of 2016.
- The total national healthcare expenditures for cancer in 2016 reached $74.8 billion.[3]

Despite these figures, our medical authorities continue to assure us that we have made significant progress in this losing war.

Deconstructing the Statistics

Dr. Samuel Epstein, chair of the Cancer Prevention Coalition and professor emeritus at the University of Illinois, Chicago School of Public Health, has been an outspoken opponent of the war on cancer. Epstein has documented the fallacies of claims made by the National Cancer Institute (NCI), the American Cancer Society (ACS), and the Centers for Disease Control and Prevention (CDC) that progress is being made. These claims, according to Epstein, are often false and misleading. For example, statistics show that cancer rates between 1975 and 2008 increased by 15.7 percent.[4] The medical establishment has attempted to explain away this increase by placing the blame upon the rise in cigarette smoking. In his book, *National Cancer Institute and American Cancer Society: Criminal Indifference to Cancer Prevention and Conflicts of Interest,* Dr. Epstein debunks this claim, noting that incidences of several types of cancer unrelated to smoking have increased to staggering levels during this same time period. Liver cancer rates, for example, rose by 177.7 percent. Testicular cancer increased by 57.9 percent.[5] Thyroid cancer rates, meanwhile, have swelled by 167.6 percent.[6]

Many of the statistics quoted by the cancer establishment have been manipulated to give the illusion of progress. In *Outsmart Your Cancer,* author Tanya Harter Pierce details six methods used by health officials to deceive the public into thinking that the war on cancer has been successful:

1. Redefining "cure" as "alive five years after diagnosis," instead of using the word's real meaning, which is "cancer-free." Under this measure, a patient could have cancer for five years and die one day after the fifth anniversary date of diagnosis but still be recorded as having been cured.

2. Altering statistics by omitting certain groups of people, such as African Americans, or by omitting certain types of cancer, such as all lung cancer patients, from their calculations.

3. Including certain cancers that are not life threatening and easily curable, such as skin cancers and ductal carcinoma in situ (DCIS). DCIS is a precancerous condition that is 99 percent curable and accounts for 30 percent

of all breast cancers. If this 30 percent is deducted from the breast cancer success stories, survival rates are much less impressive.

4. Using early detection as a means to artificially increase survival rates.

5. Improving outcomes by deleting patients from cancer treatment studies who died before the protocol was completed, even if that was on the eighty-ninth day of a ninety-day chemotherapy protocol.

6. Using a questionable adjustment called "relative survival rate" whereby a certain number of cancer victims who statistically would have died during the five years because of unrelated causes such as heart attacks, car accidents, and so on, are deducted.[7]

Nor is it true that our national battle against cancer has failed due to a lack of funding. Under the aegis of the federal National Institutes of Health, the National Cancer Institute has enjoyed more than sufficient funding from the American taxpayer since its founding after the passage of the National Cancer Act of 1971. The NCI budget jumped from $220 million in 1971 to approximately $5 billion in 2015.[8,9] Despite this increase, only a miniscule percentage of the group's budget has been spent on what should be the focus of the war on cancer: prevention. Worse, the funds allocated to help prevent this disease are drying up. In 2000, 11.8 percent of the NCI budget was set aside for prevention, and in 2015, this figure dropped to a mere 4.5 percent.[10,11]

Missing the Mark on Cancer Treatment

Not only does prevention account for a small percentage of cancer research dollars, but our national health authorities continue to downplay the risks from exposure to environmental toxins. This may be our most important area of focus for a national campaign to prevent cancer. In a 2009 letter to congressional officials, Dr. Epstein and his colleagues Dr. Richard Clapp, Dr. Nicholas Ashford, and the late Dr. Quentin Young of the Cancer Prevention Coalition (CPC) explained why progress cannot be made without an honest discussion about limiting exposure to known environmental carcinogens. Their key points include the following:

- Exposure to cancer-causing agents such as asbestos, silica, formaldehyde, benzene, chlorinated organic pesticides, and organic solvents in the environment and workplace is the largest factor contributing to the increase in nonsmoking-related cancers since 1975.
- The incidence of breast cancer has risen significantly because of environmental factors such as birth control pills, synthetic estrogen replacement therapy, toxic ingredients in cosmetics and personal care products, and routine radiation exposure from mammograms.
- Pesticides, ionizing radiation, nitrites used to preserve meats, and parental exposure to occupational carcinogens are the primary causes of the 55-percent increase in childhood leukemia.
- Hormonal ingredients in our personal care products and hormonal residues in our food have contributed to a 49 percent rise in testicular cancer rates since 1975.
- Exposure to ionizing radiation has resulted in a 116 percent rise in thyroid cancer rates since 1975.[12]

Despite the clear evidence implicating environmental toxins as the primary cause of many cancers, the NCI has consistently understated or denied this connection. According the NCI's claims, only 6 percent of all cancer events are attributable to environmental and occupational carcinogens. Further, the NCI has ignored demands from government officials and scientists to create a comprehensive list of carcinogens.[13]

Yet there is a significant body of scientific research showing the link between environmental variables and many types of cancer. In her book *Genetic Engineering, Dream or Nightmare?*, Dr. Mae Wan Ho hypothesizes that cancer is actually an epigenetic disease, a condition resulting from "a change of the cell or gene expression state in response to the environment."[14] This is in stark contrast to mainstream medicine's view that cancer is a determinist genetic disease brought on by DNA mutations within the cell. While the difference may seem minor to the uninitiated, Ho's theory challenges the core belief of modern medicine that cancer arises from mutations in cellular genes themselves. Instead, research should turn its attention to physiological stresses from environmental sources in order to find the root cause of cancer. The epigenetic theory is backed by numerous studies conducted throughout the world, including the research by Harry Rubin, professor emeritus of cell and developmental biology at University of California, Berkeley.[15] Rubin's and others' findings strongly suggest that genetic mutations associated with cancer occur *after* a cell has been transformed by physiological stressors such as toxic chemicals and ionizing radiation.[16] The evidence supporting an epigenetic view of cancer strengthens Epstein's argument that prevention should be the foremost consideration in the war on cancer.

If the NCI has adopted policies that hamper progress to defeat cancer, the nation's other leading cancer organization, the American Cancer Society (ACS), further demonstrates the medical establishment's unwillingness to face cancer's real causes.

Founded in 1913, the American Cancer Society (originally known as the American Society for the Control of Cancer) has become a prominent and influential institution in the war on cancer. Like the NCI, the ACS has ignored the connection between environmental and occupational toxins and cancer. Some of the ACS's more egregious denials of an environmental factor include the following:

- In 1977, the ACS opposed regulating hair dyes that contain paraphenylenediamine, a carcinogen known to increase the risk of liver and breast cancer.[17]
- In 1982, the ACS narrowed its definition of what constitutes a carcinogen to only those few substances that are unequivocally related to cancer in humans, contradicting decades of prior federal policy that sought to ban any food additives that were shown to cause cancer in animals.[18]
- In 1992, in spite of the scientific evidence linking chlorinated pesticides with increased cancer risk, the ACS backed the Chlorine Institute and defended its use in toxic sprays.[19]
- In 1995, the ACS published a seriously flawed study concluding that hair dyes pose little cancer risk, despite years of solid evidence establishing the carcinogenicity of hair dyes.[20]
- In 1996, along with other medical industry groups, the ACS lobbied the FDA to loosen restrictions on access to silicone breast implants, despite strong evidence connecting the gel found in the implants, as well as ingre-

dients ethylene oxide and crystalline silica, with cancer in rodents.[21]

- In 1999, the ACS dismissed the connection between genetically modified milk from cows injected with the recombinant bovine growth hormone (rBGH) and elevated breast, prostate, and colon cancer risk. Today, despite even further convincing scientific evidence, the ACS declares on its website that "the available evidence shows that the use of rBGH can cause adverse health effects in cows. The evidence for potential harm to humans is inconclusive."[22]

- In 2010, the ACS disputed the conclusions drawn by the President's Cancer Panel, which implicated environmental carcinogens such as bisphenol-A, formaldehyde, and benzene as significant factors in the cancer epidemic. The panel went so far as to admonish the ACS by calling the idea that only 6 percent of cancers can be traced back to environmental pollutants "woefully out-of-date," stating that "the true burden of environmentally induced cancers has been grossly underestimated."[23]

These are just several illustrations of the cancer establishment's refusal to acknowledge the strong science supporting a relationship between cancer and exposure to environmental and occupational carcinogens. The ACS's position is even more surprising in light of the prescient words of one of its early directors. As far back as 1937, Dr. Clarence Cook Little, then director of the ACS's predecessor, the American Society for the Control of Cancer, wrote in *Time* magazine: "Investigators have at last got a glimmering of what causes cancer. Some people inherit a susceptibility to the disease. But they do not develop cancer unless some susceptible part of the body is unduly irritated by (1) carcinogenic chemicals, (2) physical agents (X-rays, strong sunlight, repeated abrasions as from a jagged tooth), (3) possibly, biological products produced by parasites."[24]

Despite the clear evidence, our federal health officials and the national leaders in the cancer industry refuse to come to grips with the failed war on cancer. Groups such as the ACS and NCI profess to remain ignorant of the link between environmental toxins and cancer eighty years after Dr. Little made the issue public. These organizations devalue the importance of cancer prevention, manipulate statistics, and write off scientific conclusions that could protect millions of people. Why? Sadly, the orchestrators of this so-called war on cancer are not virtuous independent researchers searching for cancer cures, but a collection of well-funded special interests intent on keeping the cancer industry afloat by whatever means necessary.

Conflicts of Interest at the ACS and NCI

We don't have to look far to find heavy corporate manipulation of public cancer policy in both the ACS and the NCI. For over half a century, a collection of special interests has figured prominently in the decision-making that goes on at the ACS. Throughout the 1940s, the leadership at the ACS was taken over by a group of powerful corporate leaders. Among the business moguls who rose to positions of power in the ACS were Elmer Bobst, the CEO of the pharmaceutical company Warner Chilcott, and W. B. Lewis, who served as the vice president for tobacco company Liggett and Myers. Lewis was instrumental in suppressing a study by two researchers at the ACS showing convincing evidence of a link between lung cancer and smoking.

The ACS receives sizeable donations from corporations that either sell carcinogenic products or stand to profit from the cancer epidemic itself. According to a report by Samuel Epstein, companies that have donated more than $100,000 to the ACS in previous years include the following:

- Petrochemical companies (DuPont, BP, and Pennzoil)
- Industrial waste companies (BFI Waste Systems)
- Junk food companies (Wendy's International, McDonalds's, Unilever / Best Foods, and Coca-Cola)
- Big Pharma (AstraZeneca, Bristol Myers Squibb, GlaxoSmithKline, Merck & Company, and Novartis)
- Biotech companies (Amgen and Genentech)
- Cosmetic companies (Christian Dior, Avon, Revlon, Elizabeth Arden, and Estée Lauder)
- Auto companies (Nissan and General Motors)[25]

The influence held by special interests in dictating ACS's policy is also evident when scrutinizing the organization's board of trustees. Described as the world's wealthiest nonprofit,[26] the ACS Foundation was started in 1992 to solicit large contributions from wealthy donors. Those who have sat on the foundation's board have strong ties to different sectors of American big business. Former board members include Alan Gevertzen, the former chair of the board of contracting giant Boeing; Sumner M. Redstone, media tycoon and majority owner of CBS News and Viacom; and Gordon Binder, former chair and CEO of the world's largest independent biotechnology company, Amgen.[27]

Despite its nonprofit status, the ACS has amassed considerable wealth over the years through donations from both the public and private enterprises. In 1988, only a paltry 26 percent of the society's $400 million budget went toward medical research and programs, while the remaining funds were put toward so-called operating expenses—60 percent of which were allotted for "generous salaries, pensions, executive benefits, and overhead."[28]

The money flowing into the ACS has increased tremendously since the 1980s, exceeding $1.33 billion in 2009.[29] That same year, the CEO of the American Cancer Society, John Seffrin, earned $914,906,[30] and two former ACS officials were given even more generous payouts: the former National Vice President of Divisional Services, William Barram, and the retired Deputy CEO, Donald Thomas, earned $1,550,705 and $1,407,719, respectively.[31]

As of 2016, the well-respected watchdog group Charity Navigator, which evaluates the accountability, transparency, and finances of charities, gave a two-star (out of a possible four stars) overall rating to the ACS. In the financial category, the ACS was given a one-star rating.[32]

As with the ACS, many NCI policies have long been shaped by special interests. The NCI has a history of close ties with groups that manufacture or promote cancer-causing products. In 1971, at the beginning of Nixon's War on Cancer, the President's Cancer Panel was created to oversee the NCI as the president's watchdog. The first chair of the President's Cancer Panel was Benno C. Schmidt, partner of the wealthy Jock Whitney in one of the first venture capital firms, J. H. Whitney & Co., which invested heavily in chemical and pharmaceutical companies. In addition to having a cozy relationship with the oil, steel, and chemical industries, Schmidt served as the executive of a pharmaceutical company and was on many company boards of directors.[33] When Schmidt's tenure ended as chair of the President's Cancer Panel, he was replaced by Armand Hammer, the wealthy industrialist who presided over one of the country's largest chemical companies, Occidental Petroleum.[34] The record reflects that under the leadership of these men, the NCI prioritized the creation of ineffective, costly, and toxic cancer drugs while neglecting to emphasize the importance of prevention.

Other examples of conflicts of interest within the NCI abound. In 1992, NCI sponsored research by Bristol-Myers Squibb to develop what would become the breast cancer chemotherapy drug Taxol, which a study published in the *New England Journal of Medicine* in 2007 exposed as wholly ineffective in treating the most common form of breast cancer, estrogen receptor negative.[35] This means around twenty thousand American women are unnecessarily suffering debilitating side effects from a useless chemotherapy treatment each year.[36]

In 1995, the National Institutes of Health director Harold Varmus further opened the doors to pharmaceutical industry influence by granting NCI employees free license to consult with the drug industry. No wonder that former NCI Director Samuel Broder stated in a 1998 interview with the *Washington Post* that "the NCI has become what amounts to a government pharmaceutical company."[37]

And in 1997, drugmaker Zeneca received the NCI's endorsement for its breast cancer prevention drug tamoxifen after spending millions to sponsor the NCI's and ACS's National Breast Cancer Awareness Month. Zeneca neglected to inform women that its use significantly increases a woman's chance of developing uterine cancer.

By 2004, Leland Hartwell, Nobel laureate and president of the Fred Hutchinson Cancer Control Center, had concluded that the majority of the NCI's $4.7 billion budget is put toward "promoting ineffective drugs" for terminal diseases.[38]

Mainstream Prevention and Detection—More Harm Than Good?

Not only does modern medicine irresponsibly emphasize cancer treatment over prevention; many of the prevention methods pushed on patients by the medical-industrial complex are highly questionable. Some of the most popular treatments in use today are often unsuccessful and dangerous. While the inadequacies of conventional preventive medicine result in undue harm to millions of patients, there are several parties that profit tremendously. These include biotechnology, pharmaceutical, and insurance firms as well as hospitals and clinical laboratories.

Mammography Mendacity

We have a health-care system in the United States that emphasizes early diagnosis and treatment. On face value this sounds like a logical and prudent approach. However, testing healthy individuals for microscopic signs of illness places a strain on time, money, and resources, while the tests themselves can be invasive, harmful, and even fatal. There is perhaps no better example of this than the $5 billion[39] that American women spend annually on mammograms. Lauded as a tool that saves lives, mammograms have started to come under attack by a host of critics and consumers, with good reason. A mammogram is an expensive test that requires a slew of health-care professionals: a skilled technician to do the procedure, one or two board-certified radiologists to interpret the results, and a primary care physician to discuss the results. A suspicious finding usually requires a repeat mammogram, possibly a surgeon, a surgery suite, a nurse, an anesthesiologist to do a biopsy, a pathologist to interpret those results, and a return to the primary care physician. How many thousands of dollars does this add up to so far? And how much stress and anxiety does it create for the woman who worries about the outcome? Studies show that women experience severe psychological distress for up to a year or more as a result of a breast cancer scare.[40]

Nowhere in this scenario are women warned about the dangers of mammograms. Despite races for the cure and other relentless paid advocacy programs compelling women to undergo this painful procedure, mammograms are still a crude and inaccurate diagnostic test for breast cancer. There are large numbers of both false positives and false negatives, meaning that women will be told they have cancer when they don't, and told they don't have cancer when they do. A large Swedish study concluded that an incredible 70–80 percent of all women with a positive mammographic diagnosis of cancer were found not to have cancer on biopsy.[41] Over the course of the next decade, American women are expected to spend as much as $70 billion on unnecessary surgeries stemming from false positive mammogram results.[42]

It is estimated that for 2,000 women who receive mammograms regularly over a ten-year period, one life will be saved, but ten more will undergo needless and harmful treatment for cancer that they don't have—including chemotherapy, radiation, and even breast removal.[43] Conversely, a supposed clean bill of health from a normal mammogram result is not something that should cause any woman to breathe a sigh of relief. Many women have a negative mammogram only to discover a suspicious lump on their own a few weeks or months later.

Meanwhile, research presented at the Radiological Society of North America's 95th Scientific Assembly and Annual Meeting in 2009 incriminated low-dose radiation as a key factor in the development of breast cancer. The research demonstrated that women were 2.5 times more likely to develop breast cancer if they had received either a mammogram or chest X-ray before the age of twenty.

The breast cancer awareness industry tells us that more women have breast cancer than ever before, but the survival rate has increased because of mammograms and early treatment. We are not made aware that a significant percentage of the increase in breast cancer is due to mammograms finding cancer that isn't there, which possibly explains the improved cure rate. Nor are we made aware that the definition of breast cancer has changed significantly since the advent of mammograms. A frequently overlooked statistic shows that the rate of one type of breast cancer, ductal carcinoma in situ (DCIS), has skyrocketed by 328 percent since mammograms were first introduced in the 1970s.[44] DCIS is a condition that can only be found by mammography, because these lesions are too small to be picked up by physical examination. DCIS is currently the most common diagnosis resulting from breast tissue biopsy, but is DCIS even breast cancer at all? Ductal carcinoma in situ is actually a *precursor lesion* for breast cancer. Rather than cancer itself, a precursor lesion is a collection of cells that could grow into breast cancer, but also might not—we simply cannot know and have no way to predict the outcome. DCIS has been called the poster child for uncertainty, as it remains unclear whether the condition poses a serious threat to women's health. Studies of DCIS that were missed at biopsy suggest that the lifetime risk of progression to cancer if untreated is very low.[45]

The mammography industry is very lucrative and powerful, and has worked effectively to prevent other means of breast cancer identification from being developed. In fact, studies show that MRI would likely be more effective at identifying breast cancer, and that thermography also shows promise as a technology that is noninvasive and does not emit radiation. While a mammogram begins to detect cancer clumps of about four billion cells, thermographic imaging may be even more sensitive, picking up abnormal growth as small as 256 cells.[46] However, we must keep in mind that so-called "early detection" is a dangerously misleading term because finding cells that are abnormal is not the same thing as identifying cancer. There are many abnormal cells that never progress to malignancy, and we truly cannot tell the difference in most cases. Thermograms, like mammograms, hold the potential for disease mongering by finding abnormal cells that will not develop into cancer, thus bringing women into a destructive treatment regimen they do not need.

There is an enormous conflict of interest between our cancer authorities and promoters of mammography—no fewer than five American Cancer Society presidents have been radiologists specializing in mammography. In light of such industry influence, it should come as no surprise that the ACS has consistently adopted policies favorable to the companies that make mammogram machines, such as DuPont, Siemens, and General Electric. DuPont, in fact, was a major sponsor for the group's ACS Breast Health Awareness Program, an initiative that encouraged women to receive a mammography screenings while failing to publicize the scientifically established methods of prevention that would help them avoid the disease altogether.[47] Another disturbing conflict of interest lies in the fact that the ACS actually contracts with the mammography industry to conduct cancer research, calling the results of the research into question.[48]

A series of well-funded campaigns have prompted women to undergo regular mammograms, which are promoted as safe, responsible, and necessary. But as the Cochrane Review has concluded in their meta-analysis from 2013,

[E]very 2000 women invited for screening throughout 10 years, one will avoid dying of breast cancer and 10 healthy women, who would not have been diagnosed if there had not been screening, will be treated unnecessarily. Furthermore, more than 200 women will experience important psychological distress including anxiety and uncertainty for years because of false positive findings."[49]

A Canadian study published in *The Lancet* went further, stating that "since the benefit achieved is marginal, the harm caused is substantial, and the costs incurred are enormous, we suggest that public funding for breast cancer screening in any age group is not justifiable."[50] Despite all this, the NCI continues to recommend that all women should submit to mammograms every two years beginning at age forty. Our current promotion of "breast cancer awareness" leading to widespread mammography is simply drawing more healthy women into the patient pool rather than saving lives. Women would be better served by learning what they can do to improve their chances of never developing breast cancer. This includes eating a healthy, plant-based diet free from processed foods and animal products, exercising, losing weight, and avoiding environmental toxins that are known to cause breast cancer.

The Trouble with Biopsies

Most of us never give a second thought to biopsies. We consider them routine and harmless when, in fact, biopsies have been shown to pose considerable risk to patients. For example, studies by researchers in North America, Europe, and Asia indicate that the risk for developing serious infection from prostate cancer biopsies could run as high as 5 percent.[51] Because the prostate gland is buried amidst the intestines, the ultrasound-guided needle used in the procedure has the potential to transport antibiotic-resistant bacteria from the bowel into the prostate, bladder, or bloodstream. One Canadian study concluded that out of 10,000 men given a prostate biopsy, 9 died within a month from infections.[52] Another study published in the *Journal of Urology* in 2011 indicated that 7 percent of all men aged sixty-five and older are hospitalized within thirty days of having a prostate biopsy. In contrast, men in the same age bracket who have not been given a prostate exam were half as likely to end up in the hospital.[53] These statistics are especially alarming given the popularity of this test, which is administered to more than one million American men each year. More disconcerting is that mainstream physicians are required to administer a biopsy to make an official diagnosis of cancer.

Infection is not the only risk attached to needle biopsies. Even more concerning is the fact that sticking a needle into a tumor can cause seeding of cancer through the entire trajectory of the needle, spreading it farther and more quickly than if left untouched. A study done by a team of researchers from John

Wayne Cancer Institute in California showed that, for patients with cancer, a biopsy done with a fine- or large-gauge needle may actually increase the spread of tumor growth by up to 50 percent compared to the rate of metastasis for patients who are given more traditional excisional biopsies, or lumpectomies.

Other evidence now suggests that men receiving prostate exams are just as likely to die from prostate cancer as those who do not submit to exams. In a study published last year in the *British Medical Journal* that analyzed the prostate cancer mortality rate of 1,494 men over the course of twenty years, it was found that the "rate of death from prostate cancer did not differ significantly" between those men who were screened and those in the control group.[54] This report came on the heels of a 2009 investigation published in the *New England Journal of Medicine* in which researchers explain that only 1 out of every 1,400 men given prostate screenings would have their life saved by early detection.[55] Moreover, the study's authors noted that out of the pool of 1,400, nearly 50 of the men would end up being treated for cancer unnecessarily.[56]

A recent study on the genetics of malignant tumors has prompted many in mainstream medicine to question the usefulness of biopsies in the fight against cancer. Published in the *New England Journal of Medicine* in 2012, the study concluded what alternative health practitioners have long known—that genetic mutations can vary greatly throughout a cancerous growth.[57] The findings reveal that biopsies, which probe only a small part of the overall mass, are not always indicative of the overall genetic activity. Alarmingly, many doctors formulate treatment plans and select drugs for their patients based on a single biopsy.

Colonoscopies Reconsidered

Once considered a foolproof screening tool for potential colon cancer, the colonoscopy has shown itself to be a possibly dangerous and unnecessary procedure. A routine colonoscopy is often recommended once every ten years starting at age fifty, with the purpose of finding polyps in the colon before they become cancerous.[58] However, the polyps removed via colonoscopy are mostly adenomatous[59]—meaning slightly abnormal, but not cancerous—with no certainty of ever developing into cancer.[60]

Meanwhile, the colonoscopy procedure can be hazardous. A semi-flexible colonoscope must travel through six feet of convoluted bowel loops,[61] making four right-angle turns along the way.[62] The procedure is not always problem-free, with serious complications occurring in 5 per 1,000 US cases.[63]

Serious risks associated with colonoscopies include internal bleeding, complications from sedatives,[64] and perforation of the intestine which can lead to disability or death.[65] Additionally, excessive stress and permanent damage to the kidneys can occur as a result of improper hydration during the three-day bowel cleansing regimen prior to the procedure.[66]

The risks involved with colonoscopy have led the US Preventative Services Task Force to advise against regular colonoscopies for people ages seventy-six to eighty-five, saying that the procedure's risks outweigh its benefits for individuals over eighty-five. Researchers at Yale University Medical School determined that colon cancer tests on certain populations of ill patients may often do more harm than good.[67]

Despite these observations, costly overuse of colon cancer screenings is widespread amongst Medicare patients. While the

$2,000 operation is recommended every ten years, a study published in *Archives of Internal Medicine* revealed that nearly half of the Medicare patients reviewed had undergone a repeat exam less than seven years after receiving normal results.[68] Research suggests that hospitals, health-care practitioners, and biotech firms make untold millions each year while foisting unnecessary risk on seniors.

Conventional Treatments:
Big Money, Small Results

In conventional medicine, the usual treatment for cancer is surgery to remove the tumor, radiation to blast away tumors, and/ or administration of powerful drugs that find and kill the cancer cells. Unfortunately, these treatments are very difficult to endure and don't always work. Surgery leads to disfigurement. Radiation leads to fibrosis (scarring). Chemotherapy essentially poisons the body in order to kill the tumor. It is toxic because it introduces a poison into the body, and it is invasive because the poison aggressively invades the cells and tissues of the body. The problem is that the poison is indiscriminate. It kills not only cancerous cells but healthy ones as well. In fact, its invasion of the body is systemic (total), not local, and therefore seriously damages the immune system. Chemotherapy drugs are very toxic to healthy cells and can make you feel really sick—your hair falls out, you can't eat, you're weak, and you're deeply fatigued.

Why does the medical establishment promote radiation, chemotherapy, and surgery regardless of their poor track record on safety and efficacy? For the answer, we simply have to follow the money trail. Today, the average total cost of medical care for cancer patients, from diagnosis to death, is $350,000.[69] In some cases the cost can exceed $1 million.[70] There is no doubt that cancer is Big Business, and our costly overreliance on current treatment methods is the result of the special interests of those who stand to capitalize on human suffering.

Chemotherapy

The term *chemotherapy* refers to cancer treatment that uses strong drugs to inhibit cell growth and division. These drugs may be administered orally or intravenously, usually as part of a cyclical regimen. According to the American Cancer Society, chemotherapy drugs may be used for the following:

- To keep the cancer from spreading
- To slow the cancer's growth
- To kill cancer cells that may have spread to other parts of the body
- To relieve symptoms such as pain or blockages caused by cancer
- To cure cancer[71]

While chemotherapy manages to kill some cancer cells, a large body of research shows that the majority of patients undergoing this treatment will benefit only slightly, if at all. Chemotherapy does not kill all of the cancer cells in a person's body, nor does it prevent eventual regrowth of these cells. Moreover, the side effects of chemotherapy are often devastating and can actually promote cancer growth, including the new growth of a completely different type of cancer. By all indications, it is time to carry out a critical reassessment of this popular therapy.

Chemotherapy came into existence in the mid-twentieth century when Dr. Cornelius P. Rhoads explored the potential therapeutic use of mustard gas used during World War I in curbing cancer. Rhoads based his studies on the observations of Dr. Louis Goodman and Dr. Alfred Gilman, whose research demonstrated that the blood of soldiers exposed to nitrogen mustard during warfare had abnormally low levels of white blood cells. Because the gas was observed to retard the division of somatic cells, the researchers postulated that this toxic spray used in warfare could also be used to slow the multiplication of cancer cells. Chemotherapeutic treatment was standardized in the 1950s and has been a fixture in the mainstream treatment of cancer ever since. Rhoads, who would later become head of the Memorial Sloan-Kettering Cancer Center, was one of chemotherapy's foremost proponents.

In his book *Questioning Chemotherapy,* Dr. Ralph Moss states that only 2–4 percent of all forms of cancer are effectively treated by chemotherapy.[72] Moss writes that in the other 96–98 percent of cancers, chemotherapy fails to eradicate the disease completely.[73] A 2004 study by researchers from the Department of Radiation Oncology at the Northern Sydney Cancer Centre in Australia discovered that chemotherapy treatment contributed to the five-year survival of a mere 2.1 percent of all patients in the United States.[74] One of the major reasons that chemotherapy fails to eliminate tumors is that cancer cells have the unique ability to quickly adapt in a toxic environment in order to survive. As a result, cancer cells can mutate and become resistant to chemotherapy drugs that target a specific type of cancer cell. Despite the documented ineffectiveness of chemotherapy, the vast majority of patients are not aware of this fact. Doctors rarely share this information with patients, and statistics representing the success of chemotherapy are routinely manipulated by the medical establishment to give the appearance that it works well.[75]

Chemotherapy causes a host of acute and sometimes lethal side effects. The treatment not only eliminates cancer cells but also kills healthy, normal cells. Such toxicity leads to conditions including nausea; hair loss; anemia; permanent damage to the brain, heart, and liver; and death. The immunosuppressive effects of this treatment are significant and leave the body weakened and more vulnerable to infection and scores of other illnesses. In 2008, the United Kingdom's National Confidential Enquiry into Patient Outcome and Death (NCEPOD) reported that the use of chemotherapy caused potentially lethal side effects in 4 out of 10 patients who received the drugs toward the end of life.[76] In addition, the report concluded that chemotherapy hastened the death of 27 percent of all patients who were given treatment thirty days before death.[77]

Lesser-known side effects of chemotherapy may be equally harmful. A 2007 study published in the *International Journal of Gynecological Cancer* showed that tamoxifen, a chemotherapy drug used to prevent breast cancer in women, is associated with higher rates of uterine cancer and mortality.[78] Some newer drugs, such as Avastin, work by blocking the blood supply to cancer cells. But these drugs may also block the blood supply to the GI tract, resulting in perforation and fatal bleeding. Another study published in 2010 by Danish researchers indicated that the toxicity of chemotherapy extends to oncology nurses. The study, which examined the health records of 92,000 nurses, discovered that individuals administering and handling such chemicals were more likely to develop breast, thyroid, nervous-system, and other cancers.[79]

The financial burden of these treatments in considerable. The price of oral chemotherapy drugs, such as Avastin, Herceptin, and Tarceva, is astronomical, as the cost of some pills exceeds $90,000 a year.[80,81] When patients are insured, monthly copays are typically around $1,000.[82] Provenge, a prostate cancer medication approved by the FDA in 2010, is a prime example of gross cost ineffectiveness in cancer treatment. Prescribed only to men with "incurable" prostate malignancies, Provenge costs an astounding $93,000 a year. Much of the cost of this medication falls on taxpayers paying into Medicare, and, in other cases, the uninsured are forced to shell out exorbitant sums for a drug with very little ostensible benefit; the medication has been shown to extend the life of patients by just four months.[83]

It is important to note that the four-month survival figure was taken from a study funded by the drug's maker, Dendreon. Furthermore, the study concluded that Provenge had no apparent effect on the progression of cancer. Such contradictory findings led the authors of another editorial published in the *New England Journal of Medicine* to question the authenticity of the study's conclusions.[84]

Despite the evidence of chemotherapy's dangers and ineffectiveness, cancer patients are commonly led to undergo the treatment. The aforementioned NCEPOD report called attention to the fact that the use of chemotherapy was "inappropriate" in almost one-fifth of all cases reviewed.[85] Over the last few years, an increasing number of physicians and hospitals have revived a particularly devastating form of chemotherapy—"hot chemotherapy." The procedure combines invasive surgery with doses of heated chemotherapeutic agents poured directly into the abdominal cavity. Due to its questionable efficacy and gruesome side effects—which include death from infection and irrevocable damage to the body tissue—hot chemotherapy has been used traditionally to treat only rare forms of appendix cancer. Despite this, more physicians have begun utilizing hot chemotherapy—which can cost more than $100,000 per treatment—to treat common forms of colorectal and ovarian cancer.[86] Commenting on the growing popularity of the therapy, Dr. David P. Ryan, the clinical director of Massachusetts

General Hospital Cancer Center, stated, "We're practicing this technique that has almost no basis in science."[87]

Surgery

For hundreds of years, surgery was the only method used to treat cancer. In modern cancer treatments, the use of surgery has been grandfathered in through this history and has nothing to do with randomized, double-blind clinical trials—today's standard measures of safety and efficacy.[88] While the surgical removal of cancerous tumors is vital to patient recovery in many cases, it is imperative to shed light on the harm surgery can cause in cancer patients.

The removal of a malignant tumor through surgery can effectively stimulate cancer growth. Removing a primary tumor from the body significantly reduces the amount of two proteins known as endostatin and angiostatin from the tumor site. These proteins help regulate the growth of tumor blood vessels, and once they are diminished, metastasis can proceed at a greatly accelerated rate. This problem is compounded by the fact that surgery suppresses the immune system by inhibiting the activity of the critically important cancer-fighting natural killer cells. Not only does this inhibition promote metastasis; it can also leave patients more susceptible to infection. Compromising immunity further still are the analgesic pain medications that are commonly given to patients after surgery. Analgesic drugs such as morphine inhibit natural killer cells, which are particularly important during recovery.

A study by researchers at Memorial Sloan-Kettering Cancer Center from 2009 showed the unexpected and potentially lethal results of what we consider to be a routine cancer treatment in the form of surgery. The study, published in the journal *Cell,* examined the phenomenon known as self-seeding, in which cancer cells separate from a primary tumor and are transported to other parts of the body, only to return to the original tumor location, where they reseed themselves.[89] Through this process, chemical reactions from the immune system can trigger stray cancer cells not removed during surgery to return to where they originated, promoting the growth of another tumor. The study's findings confirm that surgery, like chemotherapy and radiation, is often neither effective nor safe, as it fails to address the root causes of cancer from a holistic standpoint.

Given the various limitations of surgery and the abundance of effective natural approaches to fighting cancer, it would seem logical to minimize the number of costly surgeries. Nevertheless, mainstream medicine readily promotes surgery even when the operation is likely to be risky, unsuccessful, or unnecessary. Dr. Laurence E. McCahill, of the Lacks Cancer Center in Grand Rapids, Michigan, found that almost half of all women who undergo breast cancer lumpectomy surgeries are unnecessarily subjected to a follow-up operation. McCahill's analysis showed that nearly half of the 2,026 women whose medical records were reviewed were operated on despite having test results showing no stray cancer cells—an indication that a follow-up surgery was likely of no benefit to the patient.[90]

A study published in 2011 in *Archives of Surgery* reviewing the outcomes of breast cancer surgeries for women in California showed that more than one-third of all mastectomies carried out were unnecessary. The findings showed that in 35.1 percent of all cases reviewed, the lymph nodes removed during the operation were not infected with cancer. Further still, the authors found that women with lower incomes were even more likely to undergo this disfiguring and invasive surgery needlessly.[91]

The *Journal of the American Medical Association* published a study that same year demonstrating that the common practice of removing malignant lymph nodes from the armpit did not improve survival rates or prevent relapse.[92] The study concluded that one out of every five women had their lymph nodes removed unnecessarily.[93] Because removing these lymph nodes damages the entire lymphatic drainage system of the arm, this surgery can result in painful cellulitis and swelling of the arms to twice their normal size. Extrapolating the data, it stands to reason that each year, 40,000 women in the United States are put under the knife. They risk complications ranging from serious infection to painful swelling of the lymph nodes, while such surgery does not increase long-term survival from breast cancer.

Radiation Therapy

About one half of all cancer patients being treated with conventional medicine will undergo some form of radiation therapy, often in combination with surgery or chemotherapy. The goal of radiotherapy is to damage the DNA in tumors by sending beams of ionizing radiation to the tumor in order to control and halt cancer cell growth. Despite its popularity as a treatment in the fight against cancer, the clinical evidence demonstrates that, in most cases, this approach to healing is not particularly safe or effective.

Much like surgery, radiotherapy was adopted as a standard practice after crude experimentation over a century ago that never proved its safety and efficacy. One of the chief pioneers in using radiation to treat cancer was the Polish-born Marie Curie. In her studies, Curie observed that inserting pellets of radium and polonium into tumors could cause them to shrink in size. Unaware of the dangers of highly radioactive materials,

Curie spent years experimenting with them, eventually becoming very ill and succumbing to aplastic anemia, a condition where the bone marrow stops producing red blood cells. Even today her notebooks are so highly contaminated by radioactivity that researchers are required to sign a waiver form in order to view them. Over the years, mainstream medicine has refined the radiotherapy techniques developed by Curie but continues to expose patients to harmful and sometimes lethal doses of radiation.

Radiotherapy causes numerous crippling side effects, including severe swelling, joint pain, fibrosis, dysphasia, infertility, stroke, and brain damage. Perhaps the ultimate irony of this form of treatment is that exposure to ionizing radiation in order to treat cancer is itself extremely carcinogenic. This is because radiotherapy not only damages the genetic material stored in cancer cells but also mutates genes in viable, healthy cells, increasing the likelihood they will later turn into cancer cells. In his book *World Without Cancer*, Edward G. Griffin writes that even though radiation manages to decrease tumor size in certain cancers, it is largely ineffective in eliminating neoplastic cancer cells, which are the true target of the treatment. Hence, radiation can often actually increase the malignancy of the tumor it is meant to control.[94]

Through statistical manipulation, the medical establishment distorts the efficacy of radiation therapy. For example, deaths from acute complications resulting from radiotherapy are not labeled as cancer deaths, but as cases in which the patient was "cured" by radiation.[95] This same misleading formula is applied when patients die from other conditions that are linked to radiation therapy, including stroke and heart disease.[96] Another deceptive tactic frequently used is claiming that patients who don't experience cancer growth within five years are fully recovered, even if the same cancer returns later on.[97]

A study out of the H. Lee Moffitt Cancer and Research Institute in Tampa, Florida, showed that women receiving radiation therapy for cancer of the left breast were more at risk of experiencing cardiovascular events such as heart attack. The study found that even ten to twenty years after being exposed to radiotherapy, women were 25 percent more likely to have coronary heart disease.[98] Another study conducted by researchers at Emory University and published in *Archives of Internal Medicine* revealed that individuals who submitted to radiation therapy as children were significantly more at risk for developing diabetes. Children who were exposed to total body radiation were discovered to be 7.2 times as likely to develop diabetes as those who did not receive radiotherapy.[99] One of the authors of the study noted, "As a result of their curative therapies, childhood cancer survivors face an increased risk of morbidity and mortality."[100]

Despite improvements over the years, newer radiation therapy technologies have been shown to damage patient health as well. A recent article written by David B. Samadi, MD, of New York's Mount Sinai School of Medicine pointed out the substantial dangers that accompany newer radiotherapy techniques practiced today. The article discusses the flaws of increasingly common treatments, such as stereotactic "radiosurgery" (also known as Cyberknife) and external beam radiotherapy, both of which involve directing a narrow beam of radiation at tumors through linear accelerator technology. Samadi explains that these blasts of radiation can result in serious damage to surrounding tissues because of excessive amounts of radiation being delivered or via defects in linear accelerators that cause the radiation to be "leaked," or directed into healthy body tissue.

These mistakes can lead to a multitude of complications, including difficulty speaking and walking, as well as ulcers, sores, and even untreatable holes in body tissue.[101] Layers of skin can die and slough off, leaving painful, ulcerated areas open to further trauma and infection. Irradiation of oral tumors can destroy the soft tissues holding the teeth in place, causing them to fall out. These forms of radiation therapy have also been reported to induce comas and even cause death.[102] It is likely that many of these destructive complications go unreported, because the damage may take several months after treatment to manifest.

An article written by German researchers in the journal *Cancer* in 2010 highlighted the sad reality of how patients are encouraged by the medical establishment to submit to damaging and ineffective radiation treatments during their final days. Despite claims that radiation can ease pain in terminally ill patients, the analysis showed that palliative radiation conferred no benefit to the majority of patients.[103] Worse still, more than half the individuals receiving radiotherapy experienced more pain and suffering as a result of the treatment, and 60 percent of the patients died while being treated.[104] In their conclusion, the authors of the study commented that such insistence on the part of doctors to extend radiation treatments unnecessarily was evidence of "overly optimistic prognoses and unrealistic concerns about late radiation damage."[105]

Investigating the economics of radiotherapy helps explain why such a barbaric treatment is possible in today's medicine. The answer, as always, is money. Radiation therapy is very profitable, despite the extra expenses for equipment, technicians, and the disposal of hazardous waste. Yet there are clear indications that many health-care professionals and hospitals look for ways to drive up the price of radiotherapy to make the treatment even more financially rewarding. A study published in the *Journal of the National Cancer Institute* in 2011 concluded that the cost of intensity-modulated radiation therapy (IMRT) for women with breast cancer was five times higher in areas where Medicare paid for the procedure.[106] In an editorial that was published along with the study, doctors Lisa A. Kachnic and Simon N. Powell of Boston University Medical Center stated that the findings "would appear to confirm the suspicion . . . that medical decision making is too heavily influenced by reimbursement rather than medical necessity."[107]

Another analysis appearing in the *Journal of Clinical Oncology* explored treatment costs of surgery and radiation for prostate cancer patients covered by Medicare. Evaluating a pool of 71,000 men between 2002 and 2005 and monitoring their progress through the end of 2007, the authors found a sharp rise in the use of more expensive treatments, such as IMRT.[108] Importantly, the more costly treatments examined in the study have never been proven to be any more effective than the less expensive alternatives examined by the team. The researchers commented that "compared to the less costly alternative, the nationwide excess direct spending for the rapid adoption of more expensive therapies was $282 million for IMRT, $59 million for brachytherapy plus IMRT, and $4 million for MIRP [Minimally Invasive Radio-guided Parathyroid Surgery] for men diagnosed in 2005."[109] In other words, taxpayers spent an additional $345 million for more expensive cancer therapies that had never been proven to be any more effective than cheaper treatments.

Our medical system's reliance on toxic and damaging cancer treatments that regularly fail to cure or help patients crystallizes one key point: the largest beneficiaries of conventional cancer therapies are, unfortunately, not the patients themselves but the physicians, hospitals, biotechnology and pharmaceutical firms, and other groups that comprise the medical-industrial complex. The unadulterated scientific evidence and statistics documenting the poor outcomes of cancer treatment should make us stop and seriously question the widespread application of chemotherapy, surgery, and radiotherapy. Even more reason to reconsider their use is the well-documented success of many alternative approaches to cancer.

The Promise of
Alternative Approaches

More and more people are waking up to the intransigence that plagues our medical system and choosing to seek out alternatives to conventional medicine, especially when it comes to cancer treatment. Today more than ever, a diverse collection of physicians, nurses, activists, and health advocacy organizations are standing up to the medical-industrial complex and calling for fundamental changes to the way health care is managed in this country.

For nearly a century, innovators and practitioners of holistic cancer treatments have explored natural and effective approaches to cancer treatment, and many have achieved remarkable results. Let's look at two areas that show tremendous promise.

The Stem Cell Revelation: Healing the Root of Cancer?

Part of the problem with the conventional approaches of surgery, chemotherapy, and radiation is that they largely fail to address the complex biochemical factors from which malignancies arise. Exciting new research into what is known as the "stem cell theory of cancer" is revealing crucial insights about how we may be able to reverse tumor growth by targeting specific types of cells through nontoxic and natural treatments.

Scientists have long studied cellular genetic mutations that lead to abnormal, carcinogenic cell growth. The mechanisms behind propagation of cancer cells are still not well understood by modern medicine. However, recent discoveries suggest that a particular type of cell called a stem cell may play a pivotal role in the development of the disease. Stem cells are undifferentiated cells, such as a neuron or white blood cell. There are a variety of stem cells throughout the body and they are essential to the formation and maintenance of healthy tissue. Operating in an organized fashion, stem cells are capable of dividing to create both more stem cells and specialized cells.

The conventional belief in mainstream medicine is that all cancer cells have the potential to grow and divide and do so randomly. In contrast, the stem cell theory of cancer maintains that only stem cells ultimately create more cancer in the body, even though stem cells make up only 0.05–1 percent of cells within a tumor mass.[110] In recent years, stem cell theory has gained traction as studies further identify the significant role stem cells played in several forms of cancer.[111, 112, 113]

Why is the stem cell theory of cancer so important? If these particular cells are indeed the driving force behind tumor growth, we can develop treatments to selectively eliminate cancer stem cells (CSCs) without harming normal body tissue. It's critical to note that chemotherapy and radiation can kill rapidly dividing cancer cells, but they often fail to kill CSCs, which divide more slowly. Why CSCs are difficult to combat with dominant conventional therapies remains a mystery. One hypothesis is that CSCs may be able to repair damage to DNA more effectively than other cancer cells. Another possibility is that CSCs possess genetic mutations that make them resistant to orthodox therapies. Nevertheless, if we accept the validity of the cancer stem cell theory, it's easy to understand why mainstream treatments are missing the mark completely.

The good news is that we already have a wealth of scientific evidence demonstrating the effectiveness of various chemical compounds—many found in our foods—to safely target and kill CSCs. Researcher, activist, and founder of the popular website GreenMedInfo.Com, Sayer Ji, has created a list of dozens of biomolecules and natural substances that have been scientifically shown to damage and destroy CSCs. Most of these substances are phytonutrients or phytochemicals, which are natural compounds derived from plants that support cellular health. Here is the list:

- 6-shogaol
- Andrographis
- Baicalein
- Beta-carotene[114]
- Blueberry
- Broccoli
- Caramonin
- Carotenoids
- Catechin
- Cruciferous vegetables
- Curcumin
- Eicosapentaenoic acid (EPA)
- Epigallocatechin gallate (EGCG)
- Feverfew
- *Garcinia xanthochymus*
- Genistein
- Gingerol
- Honokiol
- Isoflavones
- Lycopene

- Mustard oil
- N-acetyl acetyl-cysteine (NAC)
- Oridonin
- Piperidines
- Piperine
- Pterostilbene
- Quercetin
- Resveratrol
- Selenium
- Sprouts
- Stilbenes
- Sulphorafane
- Traditional Chinese medicine compound kushen injection
- Vitamin D
- Wogonin
- Xanthones

This list includes many phytonutrients that are naturally abundant in a plant-based whole foods diet. This is the same dietary protocol I have been recommending for decades to individuals battling cancer and other chronic diseases.

Questions remain about how to best target stem cells to treat against cancer. It is still unknown whether or not stem cells are found in all types of malignancies. There is still much to learn about how genes, proteins, and other biochemical agents affect CSC division. Nevertheless, the expanding body of research now demonstrates the curative properties of phytochemicals and other nontoxic substances to safely and effectively combat CSCs. Increasingly more physicians and medical practitioners are adopting these promising alternative treatments. Further acceptance of the stem cell theory of cancer could signal a positive shift in the paradigm of mainstream cancer treatments.

Later in this book we will cover the cancer-fighting benefits of phytonutrients in greater detail. First, we need to take a closer look at one compound that has been the subject of much controversy yet may be one of the most potent anticancer substances on the planet.

Marijuana as Medicine

To the surprise of many in the medical community, marijuana has emerged as one of the most exciting (and controversial) substances studied in the field of oncology during the last several years. In addition to being a popular recreational drug, the cannabis plant has been used for thousands of years as a folk remedy for a wide variety of medical conditions and illnesses. Cannabis contains an array of potent compounds known as cannabinoids, which include delta-9-tetrahydrocannabinol (THC) and cannabidiol (CBD). The potential of these biochemicals to fight disease has piqued the interest of health researchers and oncologists. Unfortunately, federal law prohibits marijuana and its chemical components from being prescribed, possessed, and sold, although some states have legalized the medical use of cannabis. Two FDA-approved drugs derived from cannabis, dronabinol and nabilone, are currently being prescribed to treat nausea and vomiting associated with chemotherapy.

Because of legal restrictions, the majority of research has focused upon cannabis's effects in animal subjects or through *in vitro* testing. Yet American scientists and researchers abroad have forged ahead to better understand how cannabinoids affect cancer in humans. Even the highly orthodox National Cancer Institute has published data on its website showing that cannabinoids do, in fact, kill cancer cells.[115] Let's take a look at some of the most encouraging new discoveries around cannabis and cancer:

- The powerful anticancer properties of cannabis extract were witnessed in a case study published in 2013 involving a fourteen-year-old girl battling an aggressive form of leukemia. The teen's family turned to cannabis extract (otherwise known as hemp oil) after her cancer was diagnosed as untreatable following nearly three years of chemotherapy, radiation, and a bone marrow transplant. The clinicians monitoring the girl found the extract to be an "effective treatment" for the disease, substantially reversing the progression of cancer in her body. The authors of the study remarked that "the results shown here cannot be attributed to the phenomenon of 'spontaneous remission' because a dose response curve was achieved. Three factors, namely frequency of dosing, amount given (therapeutic dosing) and the potency of the cannabis strains, were critical in determining response and disease control."[116] Though the girl eventually passed away, the authors concluded that her death was caused from damage sustained from her chemotherapy treatments.
- A synthetic form of cannabinoid can effectively stifle cancer cell growth and induce cancer cell death, according to a 2016 study undertaken by scientists at China's Guangzhou Medical University. Assessing the impact of a synthetic cannabinoid known as WIN55, 212–2 on a type of liver cancer, the team discovered this compound "can inhibit the proliferation of SMMC-7721

[carcinoma] cells and induce cell apoptosis [programmed cell death]."[117]

- Most orthodox physicians are reluctant to recommend alternative treatments alongside conventional cancer therapies. Nevertheless, there is evidence that chemotherapy is more potent against cancer cells when taken with certain cannabinoids. A study published in 2016 in the journal *Oncotarget* noted remarkable synergistic effects between cannabidiol and the chemotherapy drug carfilzomib. Together, they were found to effectively kill multiple myeloma cancer cells and inhibit cancer cell migration. The authors of the study concluded that "these results proved that this combination exerts strong anti-myeloma activities."[118]

- New research on THC, the compound found in cannabis that is associated with marijuana's psychoactive effects, suggests it may curb tumor growth in previously unknown ways. A team of researchers based in the UK and Spain discovered that THC shrinks tumors by triggering an interaction between two particular cellular proteins known as CB2 and GPR55.[119] While other studies on THC have demonstrated its antitumor properties, this research offers key insights into the precise pathways through which THC operates. Eventually this will lead to more effective cancer treatments in the future.

Cannabis research is still in its adolescence and there is much to learn about its role in defeating cancer. Marijuana advocates are lobbying more vigorously to fund more clinical trials on humans so that we can deepen our knowledge of cannabinoids' medicinal properties. In the meantime, cancer patients are advised to not self-medicate until more is known about how to best harness and administer cannabis.

Seeking Effective Alternatives

In light of the shortcomings of conventional cancer prevention and treatment, it's no surprise that many cancer patients seek alternative therapies in an effort to counteract the harmful effects of conventional treatment or to complement conventional treatment with therapies that may have separate anticancer effects. Using alternative approaches such as eating the right foods, exercising, attending to your emotional well-being, and taking herbal, vitamin, and nutritional supplements—these can be effective ways to enhance the immune function, reduce side effects of conventional treatment, and diminish symptoms.

To induce the body's own immune capabilities to fight the cancer is the holy grail. Remember that a normal cell has its own maintenance team that repairs damage. If that part of the cell can be bolstered and reactivated, it can do its job of overcoming the tumor-forming oncogenes, reactivating the cell's tumor suppressor genes, and subduing the cancer's growth. Whenever this occurs, the cancer goes into remission and disappears.

What can each of us do to prevent cancer and boost our immune system? Over the next chapters we'll look at five approaches to fighting cancer without radiation, chemotherapy, or surgery: (1) avoiding harmful food and toxins; (2) adopting a nutritious, plant-based diet; (3) taking antioxidants and other supplements; (4) using herbal formulas; and (5) practicing particular whole-body therapies.

Taking an "alternative" approach, of course, doesn't mean abandoning common sense. Caring for yourself properly by living a healthy lifestyle is an essential foundation. This means avoiding tobacco at all costs: lung cancer is the number-one killer of all types of cancer. It means maintaining a normal weight: being obese is harmful to the body and the immune system. It means engaging in regular physical activity: volumes of research have established that regular exercise supports the immune system and promotes psychological well-being. And it means monitoring your stress level and emotional landscape. It's been theorized that people who tend to suppress anger are more prone to cancer than others, and that people who are happier and more content with their lives tend to have less cancer and fight it more successfully. It is important to learn to release emotions in a constructive way so as not to be overwhelmed by them, and this entails addressing one's own personal needs, as opposed to living according to other people's expectations. Among those practices found to benefit cancer patients' mental welfare are hypnosis, breathing exercises, massage, aromatherapy, yoga, and positive visualization.[120]

The most important piece of knowledge when preventing and fighting cancer is this: you have control. While toxins exist in our environments, foods, workplaces, and other consumer goods, we each have the ability to take power over our own choices. With the protocols I propose for eating, exercising, and avoiding toxins, you have all the tools to make healthy, effective, and natural choices to eliminate cancer.

Testimonials

Lucinda on Advanced Breast Cancer: I had severe breast cancer that metastasized to my ribs and throughout my whole spine. My prognosis was poor. Basically, I was told there was nothing they could do for me. Still, they wanted to try by putting me through the trauma of chemo and radiation, even though it wasn't going to cure me. It could only possibly prolong my life a little bit. I refused treatment, and they just sent me home to die with a box full of drugs.

Something inside of me said, "No, wait a minute, I choose not to do this. There's some other reason I'm supposed to be here." Through the grace of God, or the universe giving me another chance, I was put in contact with a clinic down in Mexico called Genesis West. I went down in a wheelchair on just about every drug you could possibly name. I was totally nonfunctional, mentally and physically.

In the clinic I received a wide variety of treatments. A few of them involved ozone therapy and hyperthermia. Of course, diet and supplementation to build the immune system were used. The whole basis of this is that the body is built to repair itself and that it has that capability.

I came back a total fighter. Now I'm walking, talking, and living my life completely and fully. I'm fighting every day, and I'm determined to beat this.

The change is nothing short of miraculous. In fact, the medical doctors are amazed. Of course, they don't want to admit it, but it's real concrete proof for them. I haven't gone in for any tests, like a bone scan or MRI or anything like that yet, but they look at me and can see that I'm clear-eyed, walking, and functioning. Nobody can tell anything is wrong with me. Obviously, something I'm doing is working.

This experience has been a blessing for me. I want people to know that they have a lot more power and control within themselves than they know, and they need to learn that because there is always hope. You've got to always keep fighting if that's what you want.

Mike on Kidney Cancer: I'm a high school teacher from Los Angeles. In February of 1993, I had a kidney stone. After some X-rays and a CT scan, I was diagnosed with kidney cancer in my right kidney. I had two or three tumors. My doctor told me bluntly that if I didn't have a radical nephrectomy, which meant the extraction of all my lymph nodes underneath my arm all the way down to my hip, if I didn't take out my adrenal glands and kidney completely, and if I didn't have that operation by November of that year, I would be dead, no question about it. I told him that I wanted to get a second opinion, and he told me that it would be useless because it's cut and dried; there was no other thing that I could do.

My brother, Ronnie, was diagnosed as having cancer of the bone marrow by Sloan- Kettering and Johns Hopkins University. I called him to say that I had cancer, too. He told me to do what he did. He went to the Hippocrates Center and went on a fast. I went on a thirty-two-day water fast. Then I went on a seven-day juice fast. After that, I became a vegan. In other words, I didn't eat any meat, chicken, fish, or dairy products. I maintain that diet.

I go in for a CT scan every six months. The last one showed that the smallest tumor shrank a very small amount. I've had every kind of blood test and analysis that you can possibly think of. I just recently had one, and I sent it over to the Hippocrates Center because I'm going back there. They found that everything with my blood is 100 percent normal. I'm in great health.

The Hippocrates Center looks at you as a whole person. They don't threaten you; they just treat you like a human being. They use a natural diet. In other words, they don't heat anything up. Everything is a raw food and raw grains, slightly cooked.

I have maintained a phenomenal lifestyle. I'm active. I have three children. I'm not dead. I teach every day, and it's pretty hectic teaching in the *barrios* of Los Angeles. Yet I maintain a high activity in life. What can I tell you? Things look great; I'm alive, and I'm here.

1
Avoid Harmful Food and Toxins

As important as what you *do* to prevent or treat cancer is what you *avoid* doing. By now it's indisputable that you should avoid tobacco at all costs, as it clearly causes lung cancer, which kills more people than any other type of cancer. But what about other harmful substances? What foods, products, and substances have been associated with causing cancer?

The President's Cancer Panel recently took a refreshingly honest look at the link between environmental pollutants and cancer. The panel's 2010 report discussed our national officials' denial of such a connection and stressed the need for expanded federal oversight of cancer-causing chemicals used in the manufacturing of plastics, moisturizers, sunscreens, and even food. The experts sitting on the committee urged President Obama to "use the power of your office to remove the carcinogens and other toxins from our food, water, and air that needlessly increase health-care costs, cripple our nation's productivity, and devastate American lives."[121] The following pages describe some of these toxins, with particular focus on the causes and effects of our exposure to them.

Foods to Avoid

Meat

Meat should be avoided, period. The saturated fat, excessive protein, bacteria, viruses, antibiotics, and hormones in meat are extremely harmful, and this is especially true of meat from animals raised on factory farms, because these animals are given high levels of antibiotics and hormones. Estrogenic compounds are routinely injected into commercially raised animals to fatten them up. Once eaten, these hormones are stored in estrogen-responsive tissue, whether it be ovarian, breast, testicular, or prostatic, where they overstimulate the body's own hormones and lead to cancer. If you must eat meat, consuming small quantities from animals raised naturally is a safer alternative.

In 1995, the Cancer Prevention Coalition compiled a list of unlabeled and labeled toxins present in two foods regularly consumed by Americans: beef frankfurters and whole milk. While the notorious DDT has been phased out since that time, it is still found in animal products and human tissues. A growing list of studies has strongly linked frankfurters and milk with an array of ailments including colorectal, prostate, and breast cancers.[122,123]

The list of toxins in beef frankfurters included the following:

Unlabeled Toxic Ingredients
Benzene Hexachloride: Carcinogenic.
Dacthal: Carcinogen (can be contaminated with dioxin); irritant; strong sensitizer.

Dieldrin: Carcinogen; xenoestrogen.

DDT: Carcinogen; xenoestrogen.

Heptachlor: Carcinogen; neurotoxin; reproductive toxin; xenoestrogen.

Hexachlorobenzene: Carcinogen; neurotoxin; teratogenic agent.

Lindane: Carcinogen; neurotoxin; damages blood-forming cells.

Hormones: Carcinogen; feminizing agent.

Antibiotics: Some are carcinogenic and cause allergies and drug resistance.

Labeled Toxic Ingredients

Nitrites: Interact with meat amines to form carcinogenic nitrosamines, which are a major risk factor for childhood cancers.

If you do choose to eat meat, look for products that are free of antibiotics. Antibiotics not only are overprescribed for us; they are regularly injected into livestock and thus become part of the food we eat. These drugs adversely affect the immune system by diminishing white blood cells needed to fight disease.[124]

Dairy Products

Milk, too, was cited in the Cancer Prevention Coalition's list of toxins in foods. Toxic ingredients found in whole milk include the following:

Unlabeled Toxic Ingredients

DDT: Carcinogen; xenoestrogen.

Dieldrin: Carcinogen; xenoestrogen.

Heptachlor: Carcinogen; neurotoxin; reproductive toxin; xenoestrogen.

Hexachlorobenzene: Carcinogen; neurotoxin; reproductive toxin.

Antibiotics: Some are carcinogenic and cause allergies and drug resistance.

Recombinant Bovine Growth Hormone (rBGH) and IGF-1: Risk factor for breast, colon, and prostate cancers.[125]

Dairy products contain ever-larger amounts of estrogen, thanks to bovine growth hormone and the fact that we now milk cows while they are pregnant. This excessive estrogen is harmful and promotes inflammation. One reason Japanese women do not get breast cancer as frequently as American women may be that milk is not a staple of the Japanese diet. The consumption of dairy products promotes inflammation and taxes the immune system. High dietary intake has been linked with higher incidence of prostate, ovarian, breast, and other cancers.[126,127,128,129]

Poison Poultry

In the summer of 2011, an FDA-commissioned study was released showing that an ingredient added to chicken feed known as Roxarsone was contaminated with the potent carcinogen arsenic.[130] The results of the study forced the FDA to finally admit that cancer-promoting chemicals are present in animal feed. For years before this revelation, the FDA had made the erroneous claim that any arsenic in the diet of chickens was excreted through feces.[131] In reality, various levels of this harmful chemical appeared in the chicken meat sold in supermarkets across the United States and was consumed by many thousands of people. The form of arsenic found in the feed was inorganic and even more noxious than naturally occurring organic arsenic. The FDA never mandated the ingredients maker, Alpharma, to suspend sales of the carcinogenic feed, although the company opted voluntarily to do so in 2011.[132]

Arsenic-based drugs are still used today in the feed of turkeys and pigs, and we are only beginning to see their full effects. Consumer Reports recently reported that most of our domestic rice supply is now likewise contaminated with arsenic because of its presence in the animal food industry. Officials are now struggling to claim that arsenic occurs naturally in rice despite the fact that rice has been arsenic-free for thousands of years. The severity of the problem has led pediatricians to warn parents against feeding their infants rice cereal or rice milk, while South Korea has suspended its purchases of rice from the United States.[133]

Seafood That Sickens

The catastrophic offshore oil spill of 2010 poured nearly five million barrels of oil into the Gulf of Mexico. Among the far-reaching consequences of this environmental disaster were the widespread destruction of marine life and the contamination of major United States fisheries by chemical toxicants. Health safety advocates raised their concerns that seafood coming from the Gulf might contain high levels of cancer-causing polycyclic aromatic hydrocarbons (PAHs) resulting from the oil plume. In response to these worries, the FDA formulated a set of guidelines known as levels of concern (LOCs) for PAHs in seafood produced by these fisheries.

In a study published in the journal *Environmental Health Perspectives* titled "Seafood Contamination after the BP Gulf Oil Spill and Risks to Vulnerable Populations: A Critique of the FDA Risk Assessment," a research team at the Natural Resources Defense Council (NRDC) found that the FDA's shoddy risk assessment of PAHs exposed Americans to seafood contaminated with levels of carcinogens between 100 and 10,000 times what is recognized as safe.[134] The authors determined that 2 out of every 100 pregnant women who consumed quantities of shellfish deemed acceptable by the FDA would give birth to children significantly at risk of developing cancer.[135]

Processed and Other Foods

The foods mentioned above are by no means exceptional. The scientific literature indicates that consuming American diet staples, including processed foods, refined sugar, products with trans fats (partially hydrogenated oils), farmed fish, soft drinks, fried food products, and many other foods, significantly increases the risk of certain cancers.[136]

Processed foods make up a large part of the standard American diet. These foods are lacking in critical micronutrients and fiber and only impair the body's ability to heal itself. Processed products are commonly made with damaging trans fat, and have high sugar and sodium contents.

A report released by the National Cancer Institute in March 2011 revealed that childhood cancer rates shot up 9.4 percent between 1992 and 2007.[137] To account for this marked increase, some point to the increased use of toxic food additives and preservatives in recent years. The results of studies done by researchers at the United Kingdom's University of Southampton and the Center for Science in the Public Interest (CSPI) implicate common food additives and preservatives as entirely avoidable carcinogens. The CSPI's analysis found that several dyes, including the three most popularly used food dyes (Yellow 5, Yellow 6, and Red 40), were contaminated with known carcinogens.[138] These dyes are commonly added by major food producers to their products for purely aesthetic purposes. The dyes have no nutritional value yet can be found everywhere from Pillsbury

Crescent Rolls to Kraft Barbecue Sauce, Doritos, Entenmann pastries, and a broad assortment of candies.

Replace processed foods with a diet of fresh and organic fruits, vegetables, grains, beans, legumes, and limited amounts of healthy fats, with an emphasis on raw foods. When cooking, never fry foods, as this produces a dangerous amount of potent carcinogens known as acrylamides.

Alcohol

While drinking two to three alcoholic beverages weekly is considered moderate drinking in some circles, this amount has been associated with a significantly increased risk of breast cancer (one drink is considered to be 12 ounces of beer, 4 ounces of wine, or 1.5 ounces of hard liquor).[139,140]

Tobacco

While tobacco isn't strictly a "food," I'll discuss it with other carcinogens in foods as it's something we ingest voluntarily—or chew, as chewing tobacco. Everyone knows that smoking is a prime cause of the most prevalent form of cancer, lung cancer. More people are becoming aware of the dangers of secondhand smoke. Studies now confirm that 17 percent of lung cancers occur in people exposed to secondhand smoke between the ages of three and fifty but who have never smoked themselves. Cervical cancer is also associated with the inhalation of secondhand smoke. Chewing tobacco is not a good alternative to smoking, as it can lead to mouth cancer.

Toxins in the Environment

Bisphenol-A (BPA)
Bisphenol-A, or BPA, is a plasticizer widely used to manufacture food and drink can linings, plastic bottles, cash register and credit card receipts, cosmetics and personal care products, dental sealants, microwave oven dishes, medical devices, and more. While useful as a chemical that promotes smoothness and ease of flow, Bisphenol-A is an endocrine disrupter that imitates estrogen and can lead to debilitating or even fatal health conditions related to estrogen excess. The President's Cancer Panel noted that "more than 130 studies have linked BPA to breast cancer, obesity, and other disorders."[141] A 2007 review of approximately 700 studies on BPA published in the journal *Reproductive Toxicology* determined that fetuses and infants are especially vulnerable to the toxic hormonal effects of this substance.[142]

Formaldehyde
Formaldehyde is commonly found in a broad range of consumer goods, including clothing, mattresses, shampoos, nail polishes, and lotions, and is added to resins used in the manufacture of telephones and other molded appliances. Formaldehyde is present in almost all homes, as it is used extensively in plywood, foam insulation, carpeting, and other domestic materials. It is estimated that two million Americans are exposed daily to significant amounts of this substance while working.[143]

Despite its association with nasal, breast, blood, and other cancers, the use of formaldehyde is neither regulated by our government nor required to be disclosed by manufacturers. It was not until 2011 that the Department of Health and Human Services' National Toxicology Program issued its Report on Carcinogens, which classified formaldehyde as a known human carcinogen.

Pesticides

In the 1960s, science writer Rachel Carson alerted the world to the damaging properties of pesticides in her highly acclaimed book *Silent Spring*. Sadly, the world has not heeded her warning and is paying dearly for it.

Numerous studies have linked indoor and outdoor pesticide use with increases in childhood leukemia and melanoma.[144,145,146] Common pesticide ingredients such as chlordane, heptachlor, Diazinon, and chlorpyrifos are associated with lymphomas, brain tumors, and non-Hodgkin's lymphoma.[147,148] Pesticides can be avoided by steering clear of toxic household insecticides and consuming properly cleaned and peeled organic produce.

Radiation

X-rays should be taken only when absolutely necessary, as even low-level exposure has been linked to cancer.[149] The non-ionizing radiation emitted by cell phones is currently being investigated as a potential carcinogen. As a precautionary step, it is recommended to limit cell phone use. In addition, radiation from overexposure to sunlight can cause skin cancer. Wearing protective clothing, hats, and sunblock can help cut some exposure to radiation from sunlight.

Electromagnetic Radiation (EMR)

According to studies, people living close to high-tension wires are more likely to develop cancer than the general population.[150,151,152] Low-level emissions of electromagnetic radiation from these wires over long periods of time are responsible. Electrical workers have an especially high rate of leukemia,[153] as do schoolchildren whose schools are near high-tension wires.[154] In the home, EMR comes from all appliances powered by electricity, such as televisions, computers, microwave ovens, electric blankets, and digital clocks. It is therefore important to unplug these items before going to sleep if they face the bed, even when they are behind a wall.

Danger Is More
Than Skin Deep

While food is one source of unchecked toxins, some cosmetic and personal care products also contain cancer-promoting poisons. Virtually every one of them is unregulated by the FDA. There are no safety reviews carried out for cosmetic and personal care products before they hit the shelves, and companies are not required to divulge any information about adverse events that may have occurred during internal trials.

In a March 2011 article published in the journal *American Nurse Today*, Kate Bracy, MS, RN, NP, explains the FDA's inaction regarding this issue: "The European Union (EU) banned certain phthalates known to cause reproductive defects after a 2002 study found phthalates in 80 percent of the products tested. The EU has now banned more than 1,000 chemicals from personal-care products. By comparison, the FDA has banned only 10. . . . The chemical industry has strenuously resisted these efforts by lobbying and filing lawsuits in states that attempt to pass protective bills."[155]

While the dangers associated with several cosmetic ingredients have been firmly established by science, a shocking 89 percent of all ingredients in personal-care products have gone untested.[156] The sad fact of the matter is that the manufacturers of these products are responsible for policing their own goods.[157]

In 2010, the David Suzuki Foundation published a list of the "dirty dozen" chemicals added to cosmetics that damage the health of consumers. The chemicals listed that have been associated with increased cancer risk include the following:

- **BHA (butylatedhydroxyanisole) and BHT (butylated-hydroxytoluene):** Used as a preservative in lipsticks, moisturizers, and other products. Also used as a preservative in foods such as cereals, butter, meats, and beer.
- **Coal tar dyes: P-phenylenediamine and colors listed as "CI" followed by a five-digit number or Blue 1:** A ubiquitous ingredient in cosmetic products, drugs, and foods.
- **DEA, cocamide DEA, and lauramide DEA:** Used widely in soaps, shampoos, and cleansers to make them foamy or adjust pH levels.
- **Paraben, methylparaben, butylparaben, and propyl-paraben:** Preservatives present in 75–90 percent of cosmetics.[158]

The scholarly research of the David Suzuki Foundation also proves that those personal-care products that purport to be "natural" and nontoxic are often anything but. Discussing the incidence of contamination by 1,4 dioxane—a chemical that some studies have linked with cancer—the publication tells us that "in a study of personal care products marketed as 'natural' or 'organic' (uncertified), U.S. researchers found 1,4 dioxane as a contaminant in 46 of 100 products analyzed."[159]

The Environmental Working Group has established itself as a leading consumer advocacy institution. The group's website, EWG.org, offers comprehensive information on the toxicity and carcinogenicity of ingredients contained in more than 80,000 personal care products. The Environmental Working Group is a valuable resource to help consumers make smart choices when it comes to minimizing exposure to cancer-causing agents.

Testimonial

Cathy on Stage IV Hodgkin's Disease: I was in such bad shape that I couldn't lay down or walk. There was fluid in my lungs and tumors around my heart, which advanced into my abdomen. I had been on chemotherapy for about ten months. At first, the chemo got me back on my feet, but after a while it stopped working. That's when the doctors recommended a bone marrow transplant. They said it was my only hope for long-term survival.

At that point, I simply could not tolerate any more chemotherapy, and the thought of a bone marrow transplant was out of the question. I had heard about 714-X from a very well-respected physician in British Colombia, and I decided to start it. At the same time, I began to follow a holistic program.

I made quite a few changes. I had always thought that I had a healthy lifestyle, but I learned that, in fact, it really wasn't. I started doing everything that I could do to strengthen my immune system. That included a completely chemical-free lifestyle and an organic diet, with no white sugar or flour and very little dairy. The little dairy that I did have was unpasteurized and organic. I also had a lot of fresh vegetable juice and used only distilled water. I was also very careful about using chemical-free skin and hair products and about avoiding toxins such as household cleaners and pesticides. Along with that, I was on a very strict detoxification program which included cell cleanses, gallbladder flushes, and coffee enemas. I exercised using a trampoline and took pancreatic enzymes and glandulars that were specifically prescribed for me by a holistic physician. Altogether, it did the trick, and now I'm completely clear.

I began to notice improvement two to three weeks into the program. My energy level increased, and I had less pain. The best way to describe it is to say that I started to feel like my old self again. Two months after starting the 714-X, I had a CT scan done, and it showed marked improvement, so I knew I was on the right track. I was very excited. On my latest scan, which I just had last month, it showed that there was no sign of disease at all. I feel wonderful.

The most important thing is to have hope no matter what your physician tells you. You have to believe that there is more out there. You can fight for your life. I did, and it worked. It's just a matter of getting the right information. I think it's important to get information from both the medical side as well as the holistic side and find out what is best for you and what you believe in. Then go for it. Put everything into it that you can, and it will work.

2
Adopt a Nutritious Plant-Based Diet

Diet and nutritional factors are among the most important contributors to cancer development. Because so many chronic diseases, including cancer, are related to eating a diet poor in phytonutrients, fiber, vitamins, and minerals but rich in fat, processed ingredients, and additives, it is critical to consider the importance of adopting a highly nutritious, plant-based diet. Cancer has been linked to diets that are high in fats, animal products, processed foods, and even certain types of vegetable proteins. Pesticides and some types of food additives also can cause cancer. But just as a poor diet can harm you, a healthy one can also prevent cancer. What follows is a comprehensive list of anticancer foods.

Alkaline Foods

The vast majority of Americans consume too many acid-forming foods. Research has shown that tumor growth increases in an acidic environment.[160,161,162] The blood is maintained in the body at a slightly alkaline level between 7.2 and 7.4. Eating alkaline foods keeps the blood pH in its ideal range, which is important for the prevention and treatment of cancer. Ideally, the diet should consist of 80 percent alkaline-forming foods, such as those available from many raw fruits and vegetables, as well as nuts, seeds, gluten-free grains, and legumes. What follows is a list of recommended foods:

- **Fruits:** Berries, apples, apricots, avocados, bananas, currants, dates, figs, grapefruit, grapes, kiwis, lemons, limes, mangos, melons, nectarines, olives, oranges, papayas, peaches, pears, persimmons, pineapple, quince, raisins, raspberries, strawberries, tangerines, and watermelon (The most alkaline-forming foods are lemons and melons.)
- **Vegetables:** Artichoke, asparagus, sprouts, beets, bell peppers, broccoli, brussels sprouts, cabbage, carrots, cauliflower, celery, collards, corn, cucumbers, eggplant, endive, ginger, horseradish, kale, kelp, seaweeds, mustard greens, okra, onions, parsley, potatoes, radishes, spinach, squash, tomatoes, watercress, and yams
- **Whole Grains:** Amaranth, buckwheat, millet, oats, quinoa, and wild rice

- **Beans/Legumes:** Chickpeas, green beans, lentils, navy beans, kidney beans, fava beans, lima beans, peas, and soybeans
- **Nuts:** Almonds, walnuts, cashews, pistachios, brazil nuts, macadamia, hazelnuts, pecans
- **Seeds:** Alfalfa, chia, flax, pumpkin, sunflower, fennel, hemp, coconut, radish, and sesame

Other Cancer-Fighting Foods

In addition to balancing the body's pH through a mostly alkaline diet, the following foods stand out as beneficial in preventing and treating cancer.

Cruciferous Vegetables

Vegetables in the cruciferous family include kale, cabbage, broccoli, cauliflower, arugula, watercress, turnips, mustard plant, brussels sprouts, and bok choy. Cruciferous vegetables contain detoxifying compounds called indoles and isothiocyanates, which have been proven to help prevent and reverse cancer.[163,164,165,166] Recent research has identified sulforaphane, a compound found in broccoli, cabbage, and other cruciferous vegetables, as a potent anticancer agent.[167] Packed with raw and all-natural kale, broccoli, brussels sprouts, and other cruciferous vegetables, cruciferous powders can offer a rich source of anticancer nutrition.

Green Foods

Wheatgrass, barley grass, alfalfa, blue-green algae, arugula, spinach, chlorella and spirulina, and other green foods are rich in blood-purifying chlorophyll and other important phytonutrients for detoxifying the system and rejuvenating organs. Laboratory tests have established that chlorophyll inhibits the activity of carcinogens at a molecular level.[168] Studies have demonstrated the capacity of chlorophyll-rich foods to reduce tumor growth.[169,170,171] Containing spinach, chlorella, spirulina, barley grass juice powder, and fifteen other detoxifying vegetables, certain green powders are loaded with phytonutrients proven to be highly beneficial in cancer prevention and healing.

Red Foods

Research confirms that red foods such as strawberries, tomatoes, raspberries, tart cherries, cranberries, and goji berries are high in nutrients that support the immune system and fight cancer, such as lycopene and carotene.[172,173,174] Many red foods are also high in antioxidants, making them an integral component of any anticancer diet. The antioxidant power of raspberries, strawberries, pomegranate, and dozens of other nutrient-rich fruits makes some red and berry powders cancer superfoods.

Fiber

Though not a food itself, fiber is an important component of fruits, vegetables, and whole grains. The typical American diet includes about 14 g of fiber each day, which falls short of what is necessary for cancer prevention. Studies have indicated that 30 g of dietary fiber daily decrease the risk of colorectal cancer. Research has also suggested that high fiber intake may lower the risk of breast, colorectal, uterine, and prostate cancers.[175,176,177]

Olive Oil

Olive oil has been shown to possess anticancer properties. Studies have demonstrated that the monounsaturated fatty acids contained in olive oil have a protective effect against cancer growth.[178,179] Research has also shown that the phytochemicals abundant in olive oil inhibit cancer growth in vitro.[180]

But remember, more isn't always better. Olive oil still has 120 calories per tablespoon, so don't go overboard. For maximum benefit, olive oil should be used in moderation. Choose a good-quality, extra virgin, cold-pressed variety.

Juices

Freshly squeezed fruit and vegetable juices provide valuable enzymes and antioxidant nutrients that are easily digestible. Compounds in cabbage juice may have favorable effects on stomach and colorectal cancer.[181,182] Rich in beta-carotene and vitamin A, carrot juice is beneficial but should be watered down, as it is also high in sugar, and can potentially spike blood sugar levels.[183]

Green Tea

High in antioxidants known as polyphenolic catechins, green tea has been shown to help prevent skin, lung, esophageal, stomach, pancreatic, and bladder cancer in animals.[184] Studies have demonstrated that green tea extract halts the spread of chronic lymphocytic leukemia.[185] Recent research also indicates that green tea contains compounds that considerably slow the growth of cancer cells.[186]

Mushrooms

Several varieties of mushrooms have powerful healing properties. The maitake mushroom kills cancer cells by enhancing the activity of T-helper cells.[187] Research has shown that the maitake mushroom exerts a favorable effect on various types of cancer, including breast, colon, and prostate.[188,189,190] Both shiitake and reishi mushrooms have also been observed to have strong antitumor properties in animals.[191,192,193] Research has revealed that the cordyceps mushroom inhibits the division and proliferation of cancer cells.[194] And, surprisingly, the common white button mushroom has been shown to suppress aromatase activity and estrogen biosynthesis, which makes it an excellent breast cancer prevention agent.[195]

Macrobiotic Foods

Proponents of macrobiotic eating claim that cancer patients following this approach lead longer and better-quality lives. In several cases, cancer patients deemed incurable by mainstream medicine have reported full recoveries on a macrobiotic diet. Success may be due to high levels of antioxidant nutrients and a low amount of fat. In fact, the total percentage of calories from fat in macrobiotic diets is approximately 10–12 percent, a 30 percent drop from the average American diet. Best results with the macrobiotic diet are seen with endocrine-related cancers, such as cancer of the breast, prostate, pancreas, uterus, and ovaries. This is because with these cancers, too many fat cells produce or synthesize estrogen and androgen hormones that contribute to the disease; reducing the amount of dietary fat lessens hormone production.

Seaweeds

Chinese medicine has long recognized the value of seaweed for treating cancers, as it softens hardened tumors. More recently, research has shed light on the powerful mix of micronutrients, including vitamin C and vitamin E, as well as minerals, iodine, fiber, and polysaccharides in seaweed, which make it a powerful nutritional tool in combating cancer.[196,197] Considered to be among the healthiest people on earth, the Japanese consume more seaweed than any other nation.

Spices

Spices offer numerous health-promoting benefits, and certain spices have been found to aid in the prevention and treatment of cancer. Research has associated black pepper and cumin intake with a lower incidence of colon cancer.[198,199,200] Rosemary is known to help prevent DNA damage by carcinogens and suppress cancer cell proliferation.[201,202,203] Capsaicin, an ingredient found in chili peppers, kills prostate cancer cells.[204] Evidence suggests that parsley combats lung and breast cancer.[205,206]

For recipes featuring many of the cancer-fighting ingredients discussed above, see the recipe section later in this book.

Testimonials

Ed on Prostate Cancer: I had a radical prostatectomy. Afterward, my PSA kept going up. It got to 9.1. They thought it would be in the lymph nodes, and they wanted to do chemo and radiation. At that point, I was pretty disgusted; I wanted to try some alternative approaches. I went for hypnotherapy. I also started working with a dietitian to change my diet. I started eating whole foods: fruits, vegetables, foods that weren't processed. I ate more organic foods.

This was a big change for me, because I was brought up on meat and potatoes. It was also difficult for me because I grew up not liking vegetables. As a child, my mother forced us to eat what was on our plates, which included spinach and brussels sprouts and broccoli, and I didn't even like being in the same room as a brussels sprout. So I had a lot of changing to do.

I also started Essiac tea. When I started on the tea and the diet, it started moving my PSA down. It's down to 0.1 now, the normal range. I feel as healthy as a horse.

Nina on Lung Cancer: I was diagnosed with lung cancer. I was anemic and had arthritis, almost no energy, and elevated blood pressure. Pain went through me when I walked. I underwent radiation, chemotherapy, and body scans.

I was ready for a life change but was not certain where to go or whom to see. After hearing Gary Null on television and radio, I was curious and joined a health support group. I ate fresh foods and dairy.

Today I am vegan. I drink green juices and follow the protocol completely. I am cancer-free without medication. My arthritis has diminished, and I can use and enjoy my body by walking, doing yoga, and working in the wardrobe department of a theatrical company. I look forward to a good season with the crew. I am delighted with the results of each new blood test.

Karina on Breast Cancer: I was diagnosed with breast cancer two years ago, and they gave me six months to live. I did the chemotherapy. I did four surgeries, and nothing worked. I felt like I was going to die. I decided to do something different and run away from the doctors. I did macrobiotics for two years. I changed my life completely. I changed my diet. I used to eat bad food—ice cream and meat—now I eat vegetables, at least five green per day, and all kinds of supplements. I eat beans, tofu, and tempeh, and drink vitamin C. I dance eight hours per day and have a lot of energy. I still have the tumor, but it's going away.

George on Prostate Cancer: I went to a Hippocrates Health Center program for three weeks, about two years ago, and as a result of that, my prostate cancer went into remission. It was a program that consisted of organic, fresh, raw vegetables. It also consisted of green drinks, which were taken twice per day. In addition to that, there was a great deal of wheatgrass that I drank—also enemas. I did that for three weeks, and then I stayed on the program after I left the group. I went to the doctor about a week ago, and the doctor said that my cancer has disappeared; it is no longer there.

3
Enlist Antioxidants and Dietary Supplements

Antioxidants

It would be difficult to overestimate the value of antioxidants, particularly beta-carotene; vitamins A, C, and E; flavonoids; selenium; glutathione; superoxide dismutase; and coenzyme Q10, in fighting and preventing disease. Antioxidants attack harmful free radicals before they do irrevocable damage. Many clinical studies confirm their protective effects, while other research shows that antioxidants increase a patient's tolerance of chemotherapy and radiation.

Vitamin C
Vitamin C is the prime nutrient when it comes to overall support of the immune system. When fighting cancer, large quantities are required both orally and intravenously. For decades studies have

established the importance of vitamin C intake in preventing and reversing breast, gastric, ovarian, and many other forms of cancer. [207,208,209,210,211] Most people can tolerate up to 12 g daily of vitamin C taken orally, dividing this dose throughout the day. But for best results for cancer patients, intravenous vitamin C drips are needed as well. Research indicates that this method supplies the greatest healing effects because more of the vitamin can be easily tolerated. Patients are often given between 50 and 100 g of intravenous vitamin C, which is an excellent jump start to any health protocol. This treatment relieves pain and nausea, often making painkilling drugs unnecessary. High doses of intravenous vitamins C and A are associated with long-term survival of a variety of cancers, even after they have metastasized. Despite claims that vitamin C may disrupt chemotherapy treatments, recent studies have established that vitamin C kills tumor cells without interfering with the effectiveness of chemotherapy. [212,213]

Alpha-Lipoic Acid

This is a powerful antioxidant that neutralizes the hydroxyl radical (which plays a role in all stages of cancer growth) as well as other free radicals. It boosts glutathione, which combats the damaging cytokines, and regenerates vitamins C and E and coenzyme Q10. Further, alpha-lipoic acid has been shown to activate the anticancer caspase enzyme, destroy cancer cells, and help keep cancer from metastasizing. [214,215,216]

Essential Fatty Acids (EFAs)

Omega-3 fatty acids block important causes of cancer. Omega-3 fatty acids can suppress dangerous cytokines, as well as the stress-induced cytokines IL-6 and IL-10, which promote inflammation. While some fish oils are a rich source of omega-3s and have been found to reduce the risk of skin, breast, and prostate cancer,[217,218,219] not all kinds of fish are good sources of omega-3 fatty acids. It is important to know where fish came from and to avoid farmed fish at all costs.

Boosting your intake of plant-based oils rich in omega-3s such as flaxseed oil will also help you get enough of this valuable antioxidant.

Vitamin A

Vitamin A reduces infections and tumors, and is especially noteworthy for its ability to clear the lungs of smoke and other pollutants.[220,221,222] Studies of animals show a definitive link between vitamin A deficiency and higher cancer risk.[223,224] Emulsified vitamin A comes from fish oil and is easy to digest. Vitamin A also comes from nonanimal sources, such as lemongrass, wheatgrass, and carrots. Because vitamin A is fat soluble and not excreted by the body, taking too much can be dangerous; it can cause cells to swell and rupture and damage the central nervous system.

Beta-Carotene

The liver converts beta-carotene to vitamin A as needed, making it a safe source of the vitamin, especially for women of childbearing years, as no fetal problems are associated with it. (Note: People with liver problems may be unable to convert beta-carotene into vitamin A.) Studies have linked beta-carotene with a reduced risk of cervical and carcinoma cancers.

Carotenoids

Carotenoids are naturally occurring plant pigments that cause the reds, yellows, and oranges found in various fruits and vegetables. A class of phytonutrients, carotenoids have many protective health benefits: They act as antioxidants; they have strong cancer-fighting and anti-inflammatory properties; and they benefit the immune system. With respect to cancer, carotenoids are important as free radical scavengers.[225,226] Carotenoids are found not just in red and yellow fruits and vegetables like carrots, sweet potatoes, pumpkins, cantaloupes, and oranges, but also in some green vegetables such as kale, spinach, and turnip greens.

There are more than 600 carotenoids, but for the purposes of fighting cancer, three are worth noting. Lycopene is associated with lower risk of breast, prostate, lung, and colon cancers.[227, 228, 229, 230, 231]

Beta-carotene has been associated with lower levels of thyroid cancer. Lutein offers protection against breast cancer in premenopausal women.[232,233]

Flavonoids

Bright colors in fresh fruits and vegetables like strawberries, citrus fruit, and kale are usually indicative of flavonoids, which are phytochemicals that are efficient free radical scavengers. Citrin, hesperidin, quercetin, and rutin are some of these disease-fighting substances. Studies suggest that flavonoids help prevent damage to DNA, neutralize carcinogens, and lower the risk of lung cancer.[234,235,236]

Vitamin E

Much like vitamin C, vitamin E prevents cancer by preventing free radical damage and activating immune system cells to fight against tumors and infections.[237,238] In clinical studies, 400 to 1,200 IU daily have been shown to help patients with breast or cervical cancer.[239] Vitamin E works especially well when taken in conjunction with 200 mcg of selenium. Foods such as almonds, rice bran oil, kale, and avocados are particularly abundant in vitamin E.

Vitamin K

Mounting evidence points to vitamin K, a potent antioxidant with anti-inflammatory properties, as a powerful tool in the prevention and treatment of cancer. Abundant in leafy green vegetables, vitamin K has been shown to inhibit the progression of liver cancers and holds great promise for treating numerous types of cancer, including prostate and lung cancer.[240,241,242]

Selenium

This trace element, which is involved in DNA metabolism and the health of all cell membranes, has antioxidant properties, promotes cancer cell destruction, enhances the immune system, and plays a part in cancer prevention and treatment.[243,244,245] Taking selenium supplements can improve a patient's quality of life during aggressive cancer therapies.

Silibinin (Milk Thistle)

The major active constituent of milk thistle is a long-recognized antioxidant that has recently discovered cancer-fighting qualities.[246,247,248] Milk thistle is an adaptogenic herb, meaning it helps the body adapt to various types of stress and restores normal functioning. It produces repair where it's needed or shuts down cell production in tumor cells. Silibinin encourages differentiation in malignant cells, blocks the activity of the enzyme COX-2, and, by cutting off the vascular network of the tumor, inhibits the growth of drug-resistant breast and ovarian cancers.

Glutathione Peroxidase

Glutathione is found in every cell of our bodies, where it plays a major role in defending our systems. Studies show that people with lower levels of glutathione have an increased risk of getting cancer, AIDS, and chronic fatigue syndrome.[249] To stimulate glutathione production, L-glutathione and N-acetyl-cysteine (NAC, a precursor of glutathione) should be taken.

Superoxide Dismutase and Catalase

Much like glutathione, these antioxidants are frontline defenses against free radical damage, and are especially protective of the heart, brain, lungs, kidney, and liver.

Coenzyme Q10

Coenzyme Q10 works in conjunction with other enzymes in the body to optimize energy. Specifically, Q10 helps bring oxygen into the cells, acts as a stimulus to the immune system, and serves as an antioxidant, all of which are important in cancer prevention and treatment.[250,251] Studies have made the connection between Q10 deficiency and increased risk of breast cancer and melanoma.[252]

Grape Seed Extract

Grape seeds contain pycnogenol, a powerful disease-fighting antioxidant. Pycnogenol, among its various anti-aging abilities, slows cell mutations. Intake of grape seed extract has been linked with significant decreases in the risk of developing colon, prostate, and breast cancers.[253,254,255,256]

Dimethyl Sulfoxide (DMSO)

By suppressing TNF-alpha and NF-kB, dimethyl sulfoxide (DMSO) blocks the production of damaging cytokines. The combination of shark cartilage, vitamin C, and DMSO has been reported to heal basal cell carcinoma.[257]

Glutamine

Studies suggest that glutamine—the most abundant amino acid in the human body—may decrease the progression of cancer tumors.[258] It also may stabilize weight loss by allowing better nutrient absorption.

Additional Supplements

Dehydroepiandrosterone (DHEA)

Although dehydroepiandrosterone (DHEA) is naturally produced, we tend to produce less of this important hormone as we age. This decrease is connected to a number of degenerative conditions, including cancer.[259] Taking DHEA has been shown to reverse many illnesses including cancer, atherosclerosis, and diabetes.[260]

Melatonin

The pineal gland, located in the brain, produces this hormone, which not only is vital in regulating sleep cycles, as most of us have heard by now, but enhances the immune system as well. As with DHEA, levels of melatonin decrease as we age, so supplementation can be helpful. Melatonin increases the activity of our T-helper cells and aids our natural killer cells in getting rid of tumors. Supplements seem to extend the length of life, and the quality of life, in patients with inoperable brain tumors and metastatic gastric, colon, and breast cancer, as well as advanced endocrine tumors.[261,262,263,264,265]

Enzymes

Enzymes, which are catalysts for all life processes, are found in abundant supply in raw fruits and vegetables. Studies show that enzymes modulate inflammation, and that they may have a direct effect on controlling soft tissue cancers.[266,267,268] Types of enzymes needed by cancer patients include trypsin, tyrotrypsin, pancreatin, bromelain (from pineapple), papain (from papaya), amylase, and lipase. The bioflavonoid rutin may be of additional benefit when combined with these enzymes. Always consult with your physician before beginning any supplementation program.

Conjugated Linoleic Acid (CLA)

This trace fatty acid is extracted primarily from dairy products. It enhances the destruction of cancer cells and blocks the growth and metastatic spread of tumors.[269,270,271] It suppresses arachidonic acid, which triggers inflammation. In combination with beta-carotene, CLA boosts white blood cell count. A relatively small dose (3–4 g) may prevent breast cancer. CLA has been observed to exert favorable effects on colorectal, lung, and prostate cancers in animal and in vitro studies.[272,273,274] CLA should not be taken by women who are pregnant or lactating.

Modified Citrus Pectin (MCP)

Modified citrus pectin (MCP) is a complex polysaccharide derived from the peel of citrus fruits. This substance is notable for its ability to bind to galectins—the membrane proteins on which cancer cells attach in order to metastasize—thereby inhibiting cancer cells from sticking together. MCP has been shown to impede the spread of prostate and other cancers.[275,276,277,278]

Lactoferrin

Lactoferrin is a milk protein that has antibiotic properties, serves as an anti-inflammatory, and improves the immune system. It acts against the bacterium *Heliobacter pylori*, which induces gastritis, ulcers, and cancer. Lactoferrin has been observed to suppress angiogenesis and tumor metastasis in pancreatic, lung, and liver cancers.[279,280,281,282] It also binds iron and scavenges free radicals in fluids and inflamed areas. Lactoferrin is found in the milk of cows, humans, sheep, and goats and can be taken as a supplement.

N-Acetyl-Cysteine (NAC)

N-acetyl-cysteine (NAC) reduces free radical damage in the body and helps metabolize carcinogens.[283,284,285,286] This immunity enhancer also helps prevent bladder hemorrhage from cancer drugs.

Olive Leaf Extract

Known for its antimicrobial, antiviral, and antifungal properties, olive leaf extract is rich in antioxidants and is supportive of the immune system. The extract has been shown to help prevent skin cancer and induce cancer cell destruction.[287,288,289]

Shark Liver Oil

Shark liver oil contains alkyl glycerols, substances that have antitumor effects.[290,291,292] Studies show that when alkyl glycerols are given to women with uterine cancer prior to radium and X-ray therapy, the damage from these treatments is reduced.[293]

Resveratrol

This compound is one of the phytoalexins that are produced in plants during times of environmental stress, such as insect, animal, or pathogenic attack. Mulberries and the skins of red grapes are particularly rich in resveratrol. It is a very powerful antioxidant that provides greater protection against DNA damage than vitamins C or E or beta-carotene.

Resveratrol promotes healing by inhibiting the pro-inflammatory COX-2 enzyme. Studies demonstrate the ability of resveratrol to suppress tumor growth and block the formation of metastases.[294,295,296,297,298] Resveratrol has the ability to promote the destruction of cancerous cells and, by inhibiting the development of new blood vessels, reduce the volume and weight of a tumor.

Bindweed

A growing body of research points to a common garden weed, bindweed, as an excellent inhibitor of tumor growth.[299] Studies show that the anticancer proteoglycan molecules (PGMs) in bind-weed inhibit tumor growth in animals by 70–99.5 percent.[300]

Zinc

Zinc provides the body with a wide range of immune system functions. It supports the T and B cells in fighting infection and producing antibodies, and works to promote healing and reduce infection. Studies have linked high dietary intake of zinc with a decreased risk of prostate cancer.[301,302]

Chromium

The mineral acts like a hormone in the body in that it helps regulate our blood sugar levels. When blood sugar is normalized, immune function, and hence cancer resistance, is improved. This is why chromium supplements may be helpful in the prevention and treatment of cancer.

Genistein

Along with daidsein, genistein is a phytoestrogen derived from legumes that has antioxidant, anti–"bad" estrogen, and antitumor properties.[303,304]

Testimonials

Orville on Lymphoma That Had Metastasized: I am sixty-six years old and had always enjoyed good health until two years ago, when a bump appeared over my right temple. It started growing fast and was about the size of a marble. It was removed, and I was told that I had an aggressive non-Hodgkin's small cell lymphoma. I was interested in alternative medicine, and that's the route I took. First I went to Mexico for treatment, and it disappeared in about three weeks. I thought that was fantastic since I had arrived with cancer all over my body.

A few months later it began to appear again. I went to Dr. Michael Schachter's clinic in Suffern, New York. After a couple of weeks of treatments there, it vanished again.

Then it came back a third time, months later. At one point, the cancer got as large as a golf ball on my jawbone. It was pulling at my cheek and I could hardly talk or swallow. It was just a bad-looking thing and a bad-feeling thing, and it caused me a lot of pain.

This time I combined the therapy Dr. Schacter had me on with homeopathy. Basically, the therapies I used included eating organic foods and adding such things as laetrile, shark cartilage, homeopathic remedies, and a well-planned, well-thought-out vitamin and mineral program.

The bottom line is, it worked. Utilizing all the different therapies made the cancer shrink and vanish. My medical records show that it disappeared in two months and eleven days. That was a little over a year ago. Any time I get an examination, everything is clean. I don't seem to have any sign of cancer. There is nothing like the alternative way of treating cancer.

Leslie on Metastatic Breast Cancer: I have been treated at Dr. Schacter's office for a little over a year. I came from Sloan-Kettering in Manhattan, where I was treated with radiation and chemotherapy. I was there for nine months. None of those treatments worked, and the cancer kept spreading. It finally spread to my liver, and I was given six months to live.

When I came to see Dr. Schacter, I was in pretty bad shape. When I started on his oral supplements, and later on his IV supplements, I started to get better. At the same time, I cut out dairy products and red meat and increased my intake of fresh fruits and vegetables. I made sure that I had no refined foods or sugar. If I did have something it would be from the organic food shelf rather than from a fast food chain. I started juicing and that gave me a tremendous lift in energy. My body was telling me that it was very happy. That was a turning point for me in knowing how important nutrition is in battling cancer.

I started to lose the cancer from my body. The tumor markers improved, and I started gaining weight. I had much more energy. At this point in time, my blood tests are back to normal. If you looked at me, you would not know I was a cancer patient.

What happened to me is amazing. I feel that it was a combination of the right treatments for me and a lot of prayer, creative visualization, and meditation. I continue to live that way now.

Grace on Breast Cancer: The biggest change that has impacted me is that my breast cancer is now gone. There are no indications of any cancer. My vision has also improved since I started using Gary Null's Anti-Aging Vitamins.

4

Make Use of Herbal Allies

Herbs can help the immune system in three ways: they can stimulate immune defense reactions, suppress immune over-reaction, and stimulate specific functions for short periods of time. The following herbs have multiple benefits, and are particularly noteworthy for their anticancer properties.

Aloe Vera

Aloe vera is antiseptic, antimicrobial, and anti-inflammatory. It supplies the system with amino acids and minerals, such as calcium, copper, iron, phosphorus, potassium, and zinc. Aloe vera contains live enzymes, including amylase, lactic dehydrogenase, and lipase, as well as the essential fatty acids needed for optimum health. Its role in treating tumors, research shows, is due to its ability to stimulate white blood cell activity.[305,306,307]

Astragalus

Although new to the West, astragalus is a time-honored Chinese remedy. In fact, traditional Chinese medical literature from four thousand years ago says that astragalus has the ability to strengthen resistance to disease. Modern scientific research confirms these claims, demonstrating that not only does astragalus inhibit tumor growth, but it stimulates cells damaged by cancer and radiation to full function.[308,309,310,311] Astragalus is considered a life energy, or qi, tonic that strengthens vitality and increases white blood cell activity. It is safe to take on a daily basis, making it an ideal preventative tonic.

Ginkgo Biloba

This antioxidant herb, long used by the Chinese, works to counter a substance in the body called platelet activation factor (PAF), which may act to encourage tumor growth. Laboratory studies demonstrate that ginkgo may be helpful in fighting ovarian, gastric, and other cancers.[312,313,314]

Echinacea

When taken for short periods, echinacea revs up the immune system, stimulating the production and mobilization of white blood cells. It also stimulates cells in the lymphatic system, as well as important immune compounds, including interferon and tumor necrosis factor. Because of its benefits to the immune system, echinacea holds promise as a complementary alternative medicine for cancer patients.[315]

Garlic

There are numerous advantages to taking garlic, including anticancer benefits. Garlic makes cancer more recognizable to the immune system and interferes with the beginnings of tumor development. In addition, it stimulates immunity against formed tumor cells. Studies have observed a link between garlic and decreased risk of colon, lung, and stomach cancers.[316,317,318]

Research suggests that the compound s-allyl cysteine, which is found in fresh garlic, helps decrease damage to organs resulting from chemotherapy.[319]

Ginger

Ginger alleviates nausea associated with chemotherapy. It can be taken as a tea, or a small (1/2- to 1-inch) cube can be added to 10 ounces of juice. Scientific literature indicates that the anti-inflammatory properties of ginger are helpful in combating a variety of cancers.[320,321,322]

Turmeric

Part of the ginger family and an ingredient in curry powder, turmeric—or its main active component, curcumin—is a powerful antioxidant that produces a favorable effect on no fewer than ten causative factors in cancer development.[323] The compounds in this superfood have been shown to combat several types of cancer, including lung, breast, uterine, and colon cancer.[324,325,326,327,328,329,330] Curcumin inhibits COX-2 directly. It also has anti-inflammatory effects, and it is known that chronic inflammation is the cause of colon cancer. To increase bioavailability, a small amount of piperine should be added. *Caution*: This herb should not be used in large quantities as it may cause gastrointestinal distress.

Ginseng

Ginseng has a long history of use in Eastern folk medicine traditions. Studies associate the use of ginseng with lower incidences of numerous forms of cancer including breast and colon.[331,332,333] It contains ingredients called saponins that encourage macrophage (the destruction of foreign antigens) and natural killer cell activity.

Theanine

This is a component of green tea that is structurally similar to glutathione, and its presence confuses cancer cells. Glutathione acts by blocking the ability of cancer cells to neutralize cancer-killing agents, resulting in the death of the tumor cell. Animal studies show that theanine has an antitumor effect and may improve the results of chemotherapy treatment.[334,335,336]

Lentinan

This extract of the shiitake mushroom acts as an immune booster and can help reduce the side effects of chemotherapy. Peer-reviewed journals report that lentinan also helps combat colorectal, stomach, and pancreatic cancers.[337,338,339,340,341]

Essiac

Taken in tea form, Essiac is an herbal formula that has been used for years to fight cancer. Among its immune-enhancing ingredients are burdock, Indian rhubarb, sheep sorrel, and slippery elm. It is thought that the synergistic effect of these herbs may help curb malignancies.

Berberine-Containing Herbs

These herbs include goldenseal, barberry, goldthread, and Oregon grape. Berberine inhibits an enzyme prominently involved in the cancer formation. It is a potent antitumor agent because of its ability to destroy cancer cells.[342,343,344] Goldenseal should be taken for short periods of time, and not taken during pregnancy.

Feverfew

This is an anti-inflammatory herb that inhibits the production of several potentially damaging cytokines. Scientific literature has established the ability of feverfew to stem the proliferation of cancer cells.[345,346,347]

Testimonials

Marilyn on Breast Cancer: My husband brought home an article out of the newspaper about Essiac tea just before I had my lymph nodes removed. The doctors figured for sure that the lymph nodes were invaded with cancer. I started on this tea ten days before going back into the hospital. I went in and the lymph nodes and the rest of the surrounding tissues were clean. Three specialists were very surprised and kept remarking what a miracle it was because of the stage III cancer that had already broken free of the tumor and was already invading the rest of the breast.

Although I opted for a traditional approach to treatment, I attribute the lack of hair loss and the ability to handle radiation and chemotherapy without side effects to the benefits of the tea. I feel wonderful today. I've got a new lease on life. I drink the Essiac tea twice per day faithfully. This has been two years now.

Lillian on Rectal Cancer: Three years ago, I was diagnosed with a cancer below my rectum for which I received chemotherapy and radiation. That got rid of it for a while, but in time it reappeared in my liver. I received fifty chemotherapy treatments, but had I known what I understand today, I would never have had any.

I was very sick and waiting to die. I could not hold food or water down and lost a lot of weight. My bowels were totally paralyzed, and I could not go to the bathroom at all. The nurses told me I only had a short time to live, and

I wanted to die. The pain was so bad that I had to live on morphine and a narcotic pain patch.

Thank God my daughter introduced me to a homeopathic doctor who gave me a new lease on life. My doctor has done an awful lot for me. My therapy consisted of a lot of natural herbs and vitamins. I juiced and ate a diet high in healthy vegetables. Red meats were eliminated. In addition, I received colonic therapy to detoxify my bowel.

When I got home, I had renewed strength. I could walk around and even drive, whereas before I needed a wheelchair. In six months, I have been able to gain some weight back and have no more bowel trouble. I had a myelogram last month. The doctors were shocked that I was able to come this far. They can't believe it. I am a totally different person. I am amazed and my whole family is amazed as well. I feel that if I hadn't gone there, I would be gone. If I had to do it over, I would not have chemotherapy or radiation at all. I would go the homeopathic route.

Lynette on Bone Cancer: The prognosis was really bad. I went to see a bunch of specialists, and they basically all said the same thing: if I lived I wouldn't want to, because everything was just disintegrating. It was a big old mess, and I wasn't real happy because I wasn't able to get any answers.

I went to the health food store and started reading different books and talking to some people. That's how I learned about Essiac tea. I was kind of skeptical but got a number to find out what the deal was on this tea. I spoke to someone who told me that she had come across an all-natural herbal tea that doesn't affect any other medication that you're on. I said, "What the heck? I'll try it."

At the time, I could barely walk. I have total shoulder replacements and a hip replacement. The doctors tried doing bone grafts, but that didn't take. The disease was in my ankles, wrists, and knees. They wanted to do knee replacement surgery on me. In my situation, there is no stopping the disease, and there is no treatment for it. What they do is cut out the dead bone and try to put metal in there. I'm basically all bionic.

When I started drinking the tea, I could barely walk, I was on crutches, and my legs were swollen. I had them wrapped. I drank the tea three times per day. Within three to four days, I didn't have any pain.

I had some X-rays done before starting on the tea and afterward. Before the tea, they were really bad. My bones were fractured and broken, and all the ligaments were eaten away. Four weeks later, I had X-rays taken again. The doctor was amazed. The X-rays showed some bone damage, but not as much as before. A week later, I went to another doctor and had X-rays taken again. This was six weeks after taking the stuff. All the bone damage was gone. There was nothing there. They thought they mixed up my X-rays.

Today I'm great. I go biking and study martial arts. This stuff is great.

5
Practice Whole-Body Approaches

Whole-body therapies involve a combination of approaches to cancer treatment and prevention, including diet and nutrition, herbs, immune enhancement, and detoxification. The following section highlights some whole-body therapies that I have found to be safe, effective, and natural.

Gerson Therapy

An ever-increasing number of toxic substances are introduced into the environment each year, ranging from chemicals, pesticides, and drugs to the byproducts of nuclear weapons and energy. Meanwhile, new agricultural and manufacturing techniques such as genetically engineered microorganisms and food irradiation alter the food we eat in ways that have not been evaluated. Until relatively recently, the human body, which has evolved over thousands of years, seemed to do a fairly good job of adapting to changes in the environment. Within the past century, however, the rate at which people have been exposed to new and toxic substances has accelerated so rapidly that the result has been a breakdown in the body's natural adaptation and defense processes. Certain physicians view this breakdown as one of the major contributing factors to many of today's most dreaded diseases, especially cancer. The theory that cancer is triggered by environmental factors that deplete the body's natural immunity and defense capabilities is not new. In fact, the late Dr. Max Gerson took an "environmental" approach to cancer therapy more than seventy years ago. The cornerstone of Dr. Gerson's therapy is detoxification of the body through diet designed to rehabilitate the body's natural immunity and healing processes.

Although Dr. Gerson died in 1959, his work has been carried on since that time by his daughter, Charlotte Gerson. Charlotte contracted bone tuberculosis (TB) at the age of eleven while fleeing Nazi Germany with her family, but was later cured by her father of this normally fatal disease. Vowing that Dr. Gerson's work would not die with him, Charlotte founded the Gerson Institute, which operates in two clinics, one located along the western coast of Mexico about thirty minutes south of San Diego, and the other near Budapest, Hungary. Dr. Gerson was eulogized by renowned physician and missionary Dr. Albert Schweitzer, whose wife Gerson cured of lung tuberculosis in the 1930s. Schweitzer wrote in a letter to Ms. Gerson, "I see in him one of the most eminent geniuses in the history of medicine. Many of his basic ideas have been adopted without having his name connected with them. Yet he has achieved more than seemed possible under adverse conditions. He leaves a legacy which commands attention and which will assure him his due place. Those whom he cured will now attest to the truth of his ideas."[348]

The Discovery

Dr. Gerson was born in Germany in 1881. The roots of his work date to his early days as a young intern and resident before World War I. At that time, he was suffering from severe migraine headaches, which were considered incurable. After a fruitless search through the medical literature, Dr. Gerson turned to nutrition to change his body chemistry and gain relief. He was already convinced that contamination of foods by artificial fertilizers and processing had a deleterious effect on the body and felt that he might be able to improve his migraine condition by restoring normal metabolism through a healthy diet. Gerson started to experiment on himself with certain foods in a meticulously detailed scientific study. His first experiment involved consuming nothing but cow's milk. Gerson reasoned that milk, being the first food, was something that even a baby could handle, so his body should have been able to utilize it properly. But when the milk diet made his headaches worse, it occurred to Dr. Gerson that milk is not normally consumed by adult animals other than humans anywhere in nature, and that perhaps milk is a foreign substance rather than a natural nutrient in the adult human diet.

Dr. Gerson decided to conduct his next experiments using foods that were more suited for human build and body chemistry—namely, fruits and vegetables. (Contrary to popular belief, human physiology is basically herbivorous and not carnivorous. The human intestinal tract measures thirty feet in length and as such is unsuited to the proper digestion and elimination of meat, and our teeth are flat for grinding, not long, sharp, and pointed for ripping flesh.) Dr. Gerson found that he did not experience migraines when he ate nothing but grains, fresh fruits, and vegetables. He then began experimenting with single foods to discern their particular effect on his physiology. He found, for instance, that cooked foods often did not agree with him. It turned out to be the added salt, not the cooking process, that made the difference; when he ate the same cooked foods without salt, he was able to handle them very well.

Little by little, Dr. Gerson began to piece together a menu of foods that he could safely consume, as well as a list of foods that would regularly induce migraines within a few minutes of eating. He ultimately arrived at a diet very high in fresh fruits and vegetables, and freshly prepared fruit and vegetable juices, and very low in fats. Later, in his treatment of tuberculosis patients, Dr. Gerson would use a small amount of raw, fresh, unsalted butter because it is a good source of the phospholipids that form an important part of the body's defense mechanism. Otherwise, the diet was largely free of animal fats, especially cooked fats, and totally free of meats and cooked animal proteins of any sort.

By the early 1920s, Dr. Gerson had succeeded in completely curing himself of migraines with his special diet. He then started extending his findings to patients who came to him suffering from migraines. They too benefited.

Eventually, although by accident, Dr. Gerson began to use his "Migraine Diet" in the treatment of tuberculosis as well. His daughter, Charlotte, relates how this occurred:

One time, a patient came to him suffering from migraines and was given what he called his "Migraine Diet." When the patient came back after three or four weeks, he told Dr. Gerson that along with his migraines, he also had been suffering from lupus vulgaris, a form of skin tuberculosis, and that with the diet, not only had his migraines disappeared, the lupus had also begun to heal. Dr. Gerson found this almost impossible to believe, because he had learned that lupus was really an incurable condition. But there was the proof before his eyes. He saw that the lesion was healing, and he verified that it had been properly diagnosed and that there had been bacteriological studies showing that, in fact, the man had skin tuberculosis.[349]

Following this episode, Dr. Gerson was able to cure many other patients with skin tuberculosis. This therapy was later verified in large experiments in Munich, involving 450 terminal or incurable cases of skin tuberculosis treated with his Gerson dietary therapy. The treatment was shown to cure 447. From there, Dr. Gerson felt that if skin tuberculosis could be influenced by nutrition, why shouldn't other forms of tuberculosis respond? He applied this same dietary treatment to people with lung tuberculosis, bone tuberculosis, kidney tuberculosis, and other forms. One of the most famous patients he had at that time was the wife of Albert Schweitzer, who had contracted TB in the tropics. Her condition worsened when she was in a prisoner of war camp with her husband during the last part of World War I. The doctors had given up on Mrs. Schweitzer because her TB had spread to both lungs and was quite extensive. But following Gerson's nutritional therapy, she recovered and lived another forty years, until passing away at age seventy-eight.

As a result of this healing, Drs. Gerson and Schweitzer became friends and remained so throughout their lives. Dr. Schweitzer followed the progress of the Gerson therapy as it was later applied to a wide variety of diseases. When he developed adult diabetes, Dr. Schweitzer found relief through Dr. Gerson's treatment. Unfortunately, the US medical establishment has never shared Dr. Schweitzer's high opinion of Dr. Gerson. Instead of being praised, he was persecuted and harassed. Today, more than forty years after Dr. Gerson's death in 1959, his therapy remains on the American Cancer Society's list of "Unproven Methods."

The Treatment

Like other alternative cancer approaches, Gerson therapy differs fundamentally from the traditional medical treatment, in that it deals with cancer as a systemic disease rather than a localized one. More specifically, Dr. Gerson's therapy aims to rebalance and revitalize the cancer patient's entire physiology in order to rectify this systemic disorder, thereby causing the cancer to regress and preventing it from recurring.

The core of Gerson therapy is a regimen consisting primarily of a salt- and fat-free diet of organically grown fresh fruits and vegetables that are usually served raw or as juices. The primary objective of the diet is to detoxify the body and rebalance the whole metabolism, rather than simply to eliminate the symptoms of the disease. "The treatment has to penetrate deeply to correct all vital processes," said Dr. Gerson. "When general metabolism is restored, we can again influence the functioning of all organs, tissues, and cells though it."[350]

Liver Therapy

Dr. Gerson placed particular importance on the condition of the liver, which is a primary regulator of metabolism. According to Dr. Gerson, "The problem of the liver was and still is partly misunderstood and partly neglected. The metabolism and its concentration in the liver should be put in the foreground, not the cancer as a symptom. There, the outcome of cancer is determined as the clinically favorable results, failures, and autopsies clearly demonstrate. There the sentence will be passed—whether the tumors can be killed, dissolved, absorbed, or eliminated, and, finally, whether the body can be restored. The progress of the disease depends on whether and to what extent the liver can be restored."[351]

The liver's many functions, coupled with its constant interaction with the other organs of the body, give it a crucial role to play in the maintenance of health. Dr. Gerson and many other scientists have noted that in all degenerative diseases, including cancer, there are varying degrees of liver dysfunction and deterioration. Fortunately, however, the liver is not easily destroyed. While liver damage may not even be detected until liver function has been greatly impaired, the liver is also one of the organs that have the greatest capacity for regeneration. Consequently, restoration of the liver is a significant objective of Dr. Gerson's diet.

Dr. Gerson's liver therapy is multifaceted. First, animal proteins are eliminated or greatly reduced in the diet because they have been found to interfere with liver therapy and impede the body's detoxification. The ideal diet for patients on liver therapy, as mentioned above, is low in salt and fat, and high in potassium and fresh fruits and vegetables, mostly in juice form. The juice is always prepared freshly and is not mixed with other medications that could alter the pH and thereby decrease its efficacy. Restoration of the liver, which may take from six to eighteen months, depending on the severity of the illness, allows the liver to detoxify the body and produce its own oxidative enzymes.

Other aspects of liver therapy include liver injections, and lubile (defatted bile powder from young calves) and pancreatin (pancreatic enzyme) tablets. The liver injections are composed of liver extract and are given daily for four to six months. They, too, provide important vitamins, minerals, and enzymes that aid in restoring the liver to its proper functioning. These liver injections are usually combined with vitamin B12 injections, which Dr. Gerson believed are important for proper protein synthesis. Cancer patients are often unable to combine amino acids properly in order to form proteins within their bodies. Lubile was used more frequently in the earlier stages of the therapy. While it is not used for most patients today, it is beneficial in cases where the liver is extremely damaged and the bile duct system is impaired. Pancreatin tablets are given during and after the detoxification program as a backup source of digestive enzymes, because those are also deficient in most cancer patients.

According to Dr. Gerson, patients on the therapy actually begin to break down, assimilate, and eliminate cancer tumors. This is accomplished when the repaired liver is adequately producing oxidative enzymes, the general detoxification process (of which the liver is a critical part) is active, and potassium levels throughout the body are adequate.

Coffee Enemas

During the period when the body is killing, absorbing, and eliminating the tumor, detoxification is of the utmost importance. Dr. Gerson admitted that in the early stages of development, the therapy did not contain adequate detoxification techniques. "After a tumor was killed," he said, "the patient did not die of cancer but of a serious intoxication with 'coma hepaticum' (liver shock) caused by absorption of necrotic cancer tissue."[352] Thus, in addition to the other cleansing aspects of the therapy, Dr. Gerson began to prescribe frequent coffee enemas, which at the outset of treatment can be given as often as every four hours. This prescription derives from the work of two German researchers who found that caffeine administered rectally causes the bile ducts to open, instigating an increased production of bile, which flushes out the accumulated toxins.

After these enemas, Dr. Gerson noticed that patients were often relieved of pain (e.g., headaches), fevers, and nausea, which allowed him to then discontinue their pain medication and sedation. On the other hand, Dr. Gerson noted that coffee taken orally seemed to have exactly the opposite effect: it caused the stomach to go into spasm and produce a contraction of the bile ducts. Hence, while regular coffee enemas are an indispensable part of Gerson therapy, drinking coffee is discouraged.

Reestablishing Potassium Levels

Muscles, the brain, and the liver normally have much higher levels of potassium than sodium. Early in his research, however, Dr. Gerson noted that this ratio is reversed in cancer patients; that is, he found that sodium is elevated in cancer cells and that in the ailing body, potassium is often inactive or improperly utilized, or both. He felt that chronic disease is initiated by the loss of potassium from the cell system. Accordingly, another primary objective of Gerson therapy is to reestablish proper levels of potassium in the body. Because of the specific relationship between sodium and potassium, in which an increase in one mineral causes a decrease in the other and vice versa, one of the first actions Dr. Gerson advocated was the elimination of salt and sodium-rich foods from the diet. In addition, all patients on Gerson therapy immediately begin receiving large amounts of a potassium solution that Dr. Gerson developed after 300 experiments. The potassium compound he used, which is still used at the Gerson clinics, is a combination of potassium gluconate, potassium acetate, and potassium phosphate monobasic. This is administered in the form of a 10 percent potassium solution, which is added to juices ten times daily in 4-teaspoon doses. The potassium solution is never added to the liver juice, because Dr. Gerson believed that it can alter the juice's pH, thereby decreasing its efficacy. After a month, the amount of potassium solution is decreased by about half. The fluid retention and swelling (caused by a sodium overabundance) are usually the first things to disappear when patients are given high amounts of potassium in juices.

Dr. Gerson noted that even in a healthy person it is very difficult to restore potassium deficiencies. In seriously ill people, it may take as long as a year or two before normal levels in major organs are reestablished. In patients suffering from dehydration, potassium is added to the fluids therapeutically administered in the form of a GKI (glucose, potassium, insulin) solution. According to Charlotte Gerson, this solution is not specific to Gerson therapy but is recognized and utilized by the American medical establishment in general. "Dr. Demetrio Sodi-Pallares, a world-renowned cardiologist from Mexico City," says Ms. Gerson, "very much recommends this solution."[353] He agrees with Dr. Gerson that disease is systemic or metabolic. His own research in heart disease has shown that it is not a disease of the heart but a metabolic disease that must be treated with a high-potassium, low-sodium diet.[354] Dr. Sodi-Pallares found that giving GKI to heart patients with fluid retention is also very helpful. Ms. Gerson notes, "This solution helps restore potassium to the cell system. Energy is required in order for potassium to go back into the cell system, and this energy is supplied by the glucose and insulin. We use this solution quite successfully in two ways: first to replenish the patient with fluids, but also to restore potassium to the cells and reduce edema."

Diet

Every aspect of Gerson therapy revolves around the diet, which is designed to support all the other efforts to rebalance the internal body chemistry. At the clinics, all meals are prepared with fresh, organically grown produce. Nothing is canned, jarred, pickled, frozen, or preserved in any way. Between the juices and the meals, the total average intake of food for each patient is approximately 20 pounds of fresh raw food per day, mostly via juices. All refined, processed, and empty-calorie foods are avoided. This includes obviously treated foods such as white sugars and flours, and smoked, sulfured, packaged, or mass-prepared products. Other obvious prohibitions include ciga-rettes, alcohol, drugs, and caffeine, which are known to deplete the immune system and act as carcinogens. All animal proteins such as meat, poultry, and dairy products are avoided, because they are difficult to digest and hinder, rather than promote, the restoration of the liver.

Both animal and vegetable fats are also avoided, as they too can be difficult to digest and can impede detoxification. In addi-tion, Dr. Gerson found that dietary fats actually have the effect of promoting tumor growth. This accords with cancer research indicating that the higher the level of cholesterol and fats in the blood of cancer patients, the less their chance of surviv-ing. Dr. Gerson slowly eliminated all fats from the diets of his cancer patients and found that the results improved substan-tially. On the other hand, whenever he added fats (even oils that are low in cholesterol) to the patients' diets, he observed regrowth of tumor tissue. Consequently, for cancer patients receiving Gerson therapy, fats of animal and vegetable origin are eliminated as much as possible. The only exception is lin-seed oil, which Dr. Gerson found is particularly well tolerated. (For patients suffering from other illnesses, while the diet is still essentially low in fat, some raw fresh butter, egg yolks, and low-cholesterol vegetable oils such as safflower oil and sunflower oil may be eaten in small quantities.)

Dr. Gerson was a strong believer in the importance of organ-ically grown produce, and, as mentioned previously, all food used at his clinic must be grown in this manner. Chemical pes-ticides and fertilizers, he said, essentially poison and denature fruits and vegetables by altering their chemical composition. For instance, he found that many chemical fertilizers cause the sodium content in the affected foods to rise while decreasing potassium levels, which is the opposite of what the body requires to restore healthy metabolic function.

The "Healing Crisis"

A "healing crisis" is an activation of the body's defenses, and often takes the form of fever as the immune system begins to function again. Charlotte Gerson explains:

> Almost invariably, once the patient begins to produce a fever, this is followed by a tumor reduction. It seems as though the fever helps the body break down and dissolve the tumor tissue. Along with the fever come flulike symptoms such as aches and pains all over the body. This healing crisis can be quite severe in cases where the body is getting rid of accumulated heavy toxic materials. These toxins are removed through the coffee enemas, but sometimes the patient will have a very irritated colon because these materials literally burn as they are being released. In those cases, we alter from the coffee to chamomile tea enemas, which are soothing and help the body release toxic materials which have built up. We see that type of problem with patients who have been medicated a lot with tranquilizers and antidepressants. The latter are especially toxic. When they have been used a fair amount, the patients suffer a lot as they are released from the body. We have to give these patients chamomile tea enemas, peppermint tea and chamomile tea by mouth, and oatmeal gruel—all are soothing.

Usually these reactions last no longer than three to four days, and when they are over, the patients claim to be much relieved and improved, with a better appetite. Sometimes, if patients have experienced a good deal of weight loss, they become ravenously hungry. This is part of the body's normal healing process. Ms. Gerson tells of a thirty-eight-year-old patient with liver and pancreatic cancer who had been told on October 1 that she would not survive past Christmas. She was on twelve morphine tablets per day and had lost twenty-five pounds. After two days of undergoing Gerson Therapy she was free of pain and off the morphine, then went through a healing crisis with fever, came out of it after about six or seven days, and started to be very hungry. Every time she went to dinner, she took food back to her room so that she could have an extra meal or two in the middle of the night. This patient not only survived past Christmas but told Charlotte Gerson years later that she was feeling wonderful and had resumed most of her normal activities.

The Patients

Cancer patients have been treated with Gerson therapy for more than sixty years, and the results have been amazing, especially in contrast to those reported by conventional cancer specialists and agencies. The therapy was administered at treatment centers in New York and then California before the establishment of the new Gerson Therapy Center in Mexico in 1977. Currently, the California-based Gerson Institute licenses two private clinics: the Clinica Nutrición y Vida in Tijuana, Mexico, and the Gerson Health Centre near Budapest, Hungary, which opened in 2009. The Clinica Nutrición y Vida accommodates around 130 patients each year, while the Budapest clinic cares for approximately 60 patients. At any given time, thousands of cancer patients self-administer Gerson therapy at home, but the

Gerson Institute is unable to estimate how many home patients there are. A treatment at the Tijuana clinic usually lasts around three weeks and costs $5,500 per patient. The cost includes room and board for one companion to the patient.

A 2007 analysis of six case studies of cancer patients following the Gerson regimen noted that the therapy "supported patients to some extent both physically and psychologically." A study reviewing the effectiveness of treating melanoma patients with Gerson therapy compared to conventional treatments concluded that reports of five-year survival were "considerably higher than those reported elsewhere," and that "stage III A/B males had exceptionally high survival rates compared with those reported by other centers."

For more information on this therapy, contact:
Gerson Institute
(800) 838-2256
www.gerson.org

Testimonials

Tom on Skin Melanoma: In March 1982, I found a mole on the right side of my forehead. It didn't concern me much because it wasn't big; it was about half the size of my little fingernail. I talked to my family physician about it, not thinking much of it, but when he saw the thing, he was concerned. He said, "We'd better take this off and biopsy it."

They did that, and the report that came back really shocked me, because I had been eating organic foods and a right diet for many years. The news was all bad. It was malignant, it was Clark Level 4.

After the surgery, the cancer returned within ten days to the site of the incision. I guess that was because they didn't get it all. Then I began to have tumors appearing all over my upper body, chest, and arm. This all happened within a matter of days.

Initially, they wanted to do extensive surgery at the site of the original appearance, but when the thing spread, four different doctors started giving me different advice. Basically, they were all saying that nothing was going to cure this cancer.

At that point, I declined the radical surgery that they wanted to do on the side of my head, and I started looking for different approaches. I knew something about alternative methods, but nobody was at all hopeful, until we talked to the Gerson people. We called the Gerson Institute, and they said that the Gerson therapy was very effective against melanomas. They said that the fact that I hadn't had other treatments that would tend to suppress the immune system was in my favor. I knew something about the therapy, so it wasn't a complete shock. I had some belief in Dr. Gerson and his therapy, so I tried it.

I talked to Charlotte [Gerson Straus], and she said that melanoma patients detoxify rapidly. She said my chances of recovery were good, but that I would have quite a bit of nausea in the beginning. Everything she told me came true. I got quite ill initially, the type of illness that you'd have if you had a stomach flu. But I was nervous enough about my situation that after I had been on the therapy for a week or so, I thought, my God, I'm not going to be able to do this.

The family had a council of war. We all talked it over with the Institute. They calmed me down and told me they'd cut back the juices a little bit, and cut back the medicine a little for a few days, and just keep trying it. We got through that period, and I felt better again.

The heart and soul of the Gerson therapy is that every hour of the day, from eight o'clock in the morning to seven at night, you have an 8-ounce glass of fresh-squeezed vegetable and fruit juice. It alternates. Basically, one hour you have a juice that's half carrot juice mixed with apple juice, and the next hour you have green juice, which I think is three different types of lettuce, plus green pepper, red cabbage, and then apple with that also. The juices are laced with potassium salts. In addition, you have three meals. The Gerson therapy is not a fast at all, but your diet is specified.

In the beginning of the therapy, you start digesting the cancer and putting it out of the body in the form of metabolic toxins. If your body is full of cancer the way mine was, you're going to have a lot of toxins to process. To help that out, in the beginning you take a coffee enema every four hours when you're up: 6:00 a.m., 10:00 a.m., 2:00 p.m., 6:00 p.m., and 10:00 p.m. The coffee enemas put the drug caffeine directly into the portal vein. That enables the liver to detoxify a lot more efficiently than it could otherwise. The coffee enema is a great help. It relieves pain, it relieves digestive discomfort, and it is a crucial part of the therapy.

Within two months, every visible tumor on my body had regressed. They had shrunk, dried up, and fallen off. It all happened so quickly. I started out in March 1982 thinking I was a healthy guy. Then, in early May 1982, I was told that I had cancer and very little chance to live. In July 1982, I was on the Gerson therapy, and everything cancerous that could be seen had regressed and disappeared. The Gerson people said that even though everything that could be seen was gone, there was more of a problem under the surface. They recommended that I stay on the therapy for eighteen to twenty-four months, which I did. I stayed on the therapy for twenty months, and in the subsequent thirteen years, I've had no recurrence of the cancer.

Over the years, I've talked to hundreds of people with cancer of various types, and I try to share my experience with them. You can pretty much see who will succeed with this type of therapy and who will not. People used to the passive mode, where professionals do things to them—they cut, they burn, and they put chemicals in, and the patients sit there while it happens to them—are generally horrified when they find out the extent to which the patient has to cooperate in his own recovery on one of these metabolic programs. But people who can take that aboard have a very, very high success rate on this therapy. The exceptions are people who have been bombed with chemotherapy before they get on it. In order to do the Gerson therapy, you have to be motivated and open to radical change in lifestyle that a diet change like this imposes.

Joan on Breast Cancer: I had a radical mastectomy. One year later, I had a recurrence. I was not biopsied, however. The surgeon said that he would monitor this mass.

My husband and I did a lot of research and decided to try the Gerson therapy. I began the program in August 1977. By May 1978, when I saw the surgeon again, the mass was gone. Since that time, I have remained completely clear. It has been eighteen years, and I have never had any recurrences. I have had myself closely monitored over the years by surgeons and lab work.

The Gerson therapy is intensive and comprehensive. It consists of nutritional treatment through diet and thirteen juices per day. It consists of medication, potassium, niacin, thyroid, lugol solution, pancreatin, acidol pepsin, and liver and B12 combined as daily injections. It also consists of detoxification in the form of coffee enemas to help the liver. It's a very comprehensive therapy.

I still continue with my diet of organically grown fruits and vegetables. I also continue with almost daily coffee enemas. I have not eaten meat, except for poultry and fish, for these eighteen years. That was a decision I made on my own. Some people go back to their former diets, but I realized that my former diet was too high in fats and could be a possible problem again.

I did not tell the surgeon that I was doing the Gerson therapy. Nor did he ask me any questions. I wanted to keep the surgeon monitoring me, so I decided not to make him angry by telling him what I had done.

At the time, there was not the knowledge and the education about any options as far as treatment was concerned, except for the orthodox establishment options. I had been told at the beginning about the American Cancer Society's statistics and what their thoughts on treatment were. I was an RN who saw that much of this treatment was ineffective with the cancer patients, so I did not feel that the American Cancer Society was credible. Having seen this in my profession, I decided that I was going to do a different therapy. I had read about Gerson's therapy in Dr. Gerson's book. I felt it was credible and the thing to do for myself.

Patricia on Pancreatic Cancer: I had pancreatic cancer that spread to my liver, gallbladder, and spleen, and was told that I had less than three months to live. My doctors were doing nothing. They said that chemotherapy and anything else would not help me and that I should prepare my family and get my affairs in order. I was in the process of doing that. Then, one morning, my husband and I heard about the Gerson clinic in Mexico. My husband got up and said, "That's it. Pack your clothes. We're going."

We went down on March 7, 1986, and started the therapy that day. Before I started the therapy, I had been throwing up mouthfuls of blood. I was just about finished. Ten days later, I stopped bringing up blood, and the pain was gone. I said to my husband, "I don't know if I'm going to live, but I feel better than I have in a year."

Six months later, I went to see my doctor, who wondered why I was still around. He asked if I would have a CT scan, which I did. The test showed that the masses of cancer had gone. My doctor said, "I don't know what you're doing, and I don't want to know what you're doing, but just keep doing it." I think he was shocked to see that I was still around.

Another six months down the road, he asked me to take another CT scan, which I did. He said, "Patricia, there's no sign of cancer at all." That was nine years ago. Today, I feel wonderful. I have no sign of cancer at all.

I took the two Gerson books to my doctor, and he read them, but he said that it was just too deep for him. He just calls me his miracle now.

Annie on Melanoma and Cervical Cancer: I developed these conditions in 1979 when I was thirty-six years of age. My prognosis from my physicians was not good. The melanoma, in particular, was very virulent. They didn't come out and tell me how long they thought I had to live, but they tactfully tried to tell me that my chances weren't good. I read and did some of my own research and found that with stage IV melanoma, the patient tends to expire in one to five years. It's now been fifteen years. I'm not a typical patient.

I did a lot of research and picked Dr. Max Gerson's therapy because I felt that it was the hardest and the most curative. It had the best results with melanoma. I was inspired by the fact that Dr. Gerson had worked with Albert Schweitzer, and that he was a pioneer. He just was an incredible physician with a wonderful answer, but not many people were willing to use his therapy for their problems.

I found that after the first six months of the therapy, I began to feel really normal. I didn't have reactions and feelings that come when you do a metabolic therapy. I started to feel intuitively that I wasn't going to die—that I was never going to have a recurrence. I know that the mind has a great deal to do with healing. I just knew because this diet was building my cells that my mind was stronger. I felt that I had turned the corner. It's been almost sixteen years, and I feel better than I ever have in my life. I attribute that to Dr. Gerson's work and, of course, my participating in it.

Sharon on Non-Hodgkin's Lymphoma: I did not have chemotherapy. I went directly to the Gerson Hospital. I was there for two weeks, and in five days I lost twenty-eight pounds of fluid. I had been very swollen with edema. When I got back, I continued on the therapy, and in six months I went back to the doctor. I had an MRI, and my tumor was gone. I am not on a modified therapy. It's been three years.

Harold on Pancreatic Cancer: I went to the Gerson therapy center in February 1983. Prior to going there, my wife and I were on the way to Hawaii. We were in Seattle and preparing to leave for Hawaii the next morning. I got very sick and had a lot of pain in my stomach and back. We phoned the doctor who was listed in the hotel directory, and took a taxi to the hospital. I had a blood test, an X-ray, and an examination by a doctor there. The doctor said that he wasn't sure what the problem was, but he suggested that we not go to Hawaii. He said we should go home instead and get further tests done. That's what we did.

My doctor sent me to a specialist in Victoria. I went through a lot of tests that I had never heard of before. On January 21, the specialist took some blood tests and said that the amylase in my blood was high. A normal level was between 70 and 320, and mine was 627. It proved that there was a very bad infection in my body.

I finally took a CT scan, which showed a mass in the head of the pancreas. The specialist said that there was absolutely no question about it. I had cancer of the pancreas.

We had heard about Gerson's therapy through somebody my daughter knew. We phoned the Gerson Institute and went down there in February 1983. We spent one month there.

Afterward, we stayed in our condo in Escondido for eight months, because that was the only place we could get organic foods. We had our organic vegetables delivered by a lady who got her vegetables from the same source as the Gersons.

When we came home, I had put weight on, and I felt good. My blood tests were also good. I took another CT scan, and it showed no tumor. I phoned the head doctor at Gerson's in April 1984, and he told me to stay another four months on the program. That was eleven years ago, and I have had absolutely no problem since.

The Issels Treatment

Trained as a traditional surgeon, the late German physician Dr. Joseph Issels was widely regarded as the father of integrative medicine, combining alternative and complementary medicine decades before its current popularity. Issels became aware of the limitations of orthodox therapy when he began treating cancer patients and found that the survival rate was frustratingly low. His observations convinced him that the successful treatment of cancer required a return to the whole-body (or *Ganzheit*) approach to the disease. Issels strongly believed that "cancer is not just a local disease confined to the particular place in the body where the tumor manifests itself but is a general disease of the whole body."[355] Convinced of the body's inherent ability to heal itself, Dr. Issels developed a broad-spectrum therapy to restore and regenerate the body's natural defense mechanisms, which complements traditional Western medical treatment directed at the elimination of a localized tumor. With this approach, Dr. Issels achieved a degree of success in treating his cancer patients that is unparalleled in traditional medicine, ultimately demonstrating the most successful results ever achieved with late-stage cancer patients—a 16.6 percent five-year survival rate and 15 percent fifteen-year survival rate.

The Discovery
How did it all begin? In his early years of medicine, Dr. Issels put some of his theories into practice in what he would later call a *"Ganzheit"* or "whole-body" approach to healing. He required

that his patients have infected teeth or tonsils removed, because he strongly believed that chronic bacterial infection can release poisons into the body that lower natural resistance and trigger disease. Proper diet was also considered critical. The usual foodstuffs had to be replaced with nutrient-rich ones adjusted to fit the organic conditions of individual patients, but all diets were based on whole, organic plant foods. Chronically ill patients usually had to receive lactobacillus acidophilus, a cultured milk product that served as a ferment substitute to compensate for a loss of efficiency in their digestive systems. Tobacco, alcohol, coffee, tea, and other substances the doctor considered harmful were banned. Whenever possible, longstanding emotional stress was relieved or eliminated. In the meantime, the doctor went ahead with treatment of the particular diseased organ, confident that he was also addressing the root cause of the patient's sickness.

Initially, Issels's success at curing cancer or achieving long-term remission was not great. He knew that his colleagues were equally baffled by the disease, but that knowledge did not ease his frustration. Surgery and radiation seemed to bring temporary improvement, but it was clear that they did not get at the cause of the cancer and could not protect the patient from further occurrences. Surely, Dr. Issels thought, there had to be a way of applying the principles of *Ganzheit* therapy to the treatment of cancer to produce not just remissions but genuine cures. There had to be an alternative to disfiguring surgery, toxic chemicals, and poisonous radiation.

After continued experimentation, Dr. Issels began getting remarkable results with a combination of *Ganzheit* therapy, homeopathy, dietary control, and other therapeutic techniques. His practice became the largest in town, but because of his compassion for cancer sufferers and a willingness to provide treatment for low or no cost, the practice did not make him a rich man.

Using History as a Guide

Dr. Issels's antipathy toward cancer in his early years became almost an obsession with the disease. He read everything he could find on cancer and in the process became an expert in medical history. He discovered to his surprise that cancer, contrary to popular opinion, was not a modern affliction but had been observed by Chinese and Sumerian physicians and described in manuscripts dating back to 3,000 years BCE. Even that long ago, cancer was thought to result from a malfunction in the body's regulatory mechanisms and was treated with acupuncture and drugs.

Hippocrates (460–377 BCE), the founder of Western medicine, was the first to use the word "carcinoma" in referring to malignant tumors, which he believed arose from a "separation of the humors" (blood, bile, and phlegm) and was to be treated with surgery and drugs. But what Dr. Issels found especially noteworthy was Hippocrates's recommendation that the entire body be detoxified and that cancer patients be put on a special diet, much like his own *Ganzheit* theory. Further research showed that for the ancient Greeks, *diata,* or "diet," referred to far more than what a patient was to eat or drink. The term was closer in meaning to "way of life" or "lifestyle" and strongly suggested abstinence from anything that might be spiritually as well as physically harmful.

The Greek physician Galen (129–216 CE), the founder of scientific physiology, had also turned his attention to cancer, as Dr. Issels discovered. Galen also held the opinion that cancer is a disease of the entire body, not confined to the site of the tumor.

Moving forward in time, Dr. Issels read about the Renaissance doctor Paracelsus, who also felt that the physician's role in treating cancer and other diseases was not to interfere with the body but rather to stimulate the healing processes nature had provided to correct the imbalances in the body that result from illness. Dr. Issels also encountered the pioneer surgeon Ambroise Paré, who shared Paracelsus's view of cancer as a disease of the entire body, and the French thinker René Descartes, who thought cancer was caused by abnormalities in the lymph glands. He pored over the work of Percival Potts, the eighteenth-century British physician who was among the first to describe cancer as an "occupational" malignancy when he noticed an abnormally high rate of cancer of the scrotum in young chimney sweeps. In short, no one who might have something useful to say about cancer escaped Issels's scrutiny.

The work of Dr. Edward Jenner, the English physician who had developed a vaccination and checked the scourge of smallpox, seemed to offer special promise in regard to both theory and practice. Although Dr. Jenner had not been successful in treating cancer, he had produced vaccines that had shown promising results against other disorders. Equally important for Dr. Issels, his British predecessor believed that cancer stemmed from inadequacies in the immune mechanisms and that it could have a fatal effect only when the body's natural immunity had broken down completely.

Searching for a Vaccine

Following this line of thought, Dr. Issels searched for a vaccine that would bolster the body's immune system to the point where it could fight back successfully against cancer. Neoblastine, a vaccine he developed by culturing cancer tissues in a controlled medium for many times over a long period to ensure safety, seemed to offer some promise. After testing the vaccine on laboratory animals, he tried it on a terminally ill lung cancer patient, together with his *Ganzheit* therapy involving extraction of infected teeth and tonsils, and strict dietary control.

Although the patient lived three months longer than expected, the results were ambiguous, because there had been no cure and it was impossible to attribute the patient's improvement to any single factor in the treatment.

Issels became convinced that a tumor was merely a late-stage symptom, accidentally triggered but able to grow only in what he described as a "tumor milieu," the result of prior damage to organs and organ systems, especially those involved in maintaining the body's resistance to disease. The disease would never gain a foothold unless the body's defenses were depleted. Issels posited that once cancer had gained a foothold, conventional treatments could usually provide only temporary relief. While surgery, by removing large masses of tumor, might stimulate the immune system to regenerate, it was not likely to provide a cure by itself because the operation could not get at the underlying cause of the cancer. Radiation and chemotherapy, while initially successful, frequently provided only temporary relief. Nonetheless, Dr. Issels did not offer *Ganzheit* therapy as a substitute for the usual treatments, but as a supplement that he believed would make the conventional therapies more effective by rehabilitating the entire patient instead of just attacking the tumor.

Combining Traditional and Unconventional Methods

As the number of his cancer patients continued to grow, Dr. Issels began specializing in that disease. In 1950, he took charge of a thirty-bed cancer unit at a clinic in a small town in Bavaria. There, he put in seventeen-hour days, treating patients with a combination of traditional and unconventional methods. Surgery was used to remove large tumors. Drugs were administered to improve the functioning of various organs, especially the liver and kidneys, which usually are severely damaged in advanced cancer patients. The body was detoxified through the use of purifying drugs; mild purgatives; a diet high in fruit, vegetables, and grains; and the consumption of large amounts of water, juice, and herbal teas. Homeopathic remedies were used along with vaccines to stimulate antibody production.

Dr. Issels's treatment did not cure all cancer patients, but considering most of his patients were late- or end-stage in their disease, it was remarkable that he was able to extend the lives of many by months or years. Those who came to him were patients other physicians had given up on. For them, Dr. Issels offered the proverbial "last, best hope" of staying alive, a hope he was sometimes able to fulfill in ways that bordered on the miraculous.

The Treatment

Although about 90 percent of the patients he saw had already been deemed incurable and beyond the help of orthodox medicine, Dr. Issels continued conventional treatment if it was possible and appropriate. He viewed *Ganzheit* therapy as a supplement to make these treatments more effective rather than as a substitute for them. His approach added six components to conventional treatment:

- Tonsillectomy and extraction of infected teeth
- Diet and nutrition
- Psychotherapy
- Immunotherapy
- Ozone therapy
- Fever induction

Under *Ganzheit* therapy, patients part with infected teeth and tonsils. Dr. Issels viewed these as sites of infection that place an unnecessary burden on the immune system and act to lower the body's general defenses against disease. Dental amalgams also are removed to reduce exposure to mercury.

Diet is a critical component of *Ganzheit* therapy. Most meats are avoided, because meat is difficult for advanced cancer patients to digest and is usually filled with hormones, antibiotics, and pesticides that place further strain on the body. The recommended diet is primarily vegetarian, focusing on organically grown whole grains, fruits, and vegetables, supplemented by enzymes, minerals, and vitamins, with emphasis on vitamins A, B-complex, C, and E. Yogurt and acidophilus supplements are used to eliminate abnormal intestinal flora. Serum activator is administered to bring the metabolism of red blood cells up to normal levels, allowing the release of additional hemoglobin and thus increasing the supply of oxygen to the body's cells. Organ extracts are supplied to help repair secondary damage to organs and improve their functioning, while a high fluid intake backed up with herbal extracts is used to detoxify the body; improve kidney, lymph, and liver functions; and bolster the excretory systems.

Because *Ganzheit* therapy entails the treatment of the entire patient, individual and group psychotherapy is an important element. Through this treatment, Dr. Issels hoped not only to help the patient come to terms with the disease but also to alleviate or remove the psychic stress that he felt could help bring on cancer and hinder its cure.

Another major component of the treatment is a highly sophisticated form of immunotherapy, geared specifically to fighting cancer and supported, where necessary, by surgery, radiation, and chemotherapy. This immunotherapy involves a twofold approach: specific immunization against the particular type of cancer and a general effort to augment the body's natural immune responses.

"Specific immunization works on a well-tried principle," Dr. Issels wrote in his 1975 book, *Cancer: A Second Opinion.* "Once a particular cancer antigen has been identified, it is administered under conditions most favorable for the induction of an immune response that will destroy cancer cells bearing that antigen. This is really no more than an extension of the standard vaccination technique against any infectious disease."

For specific immunization against the tumor, Dr. Issels often administered a vaccine developed by Viennese scientist Dr. Franz Gerlach that was shown to cause regression of malignant tumors. Other tumor-specific immunizations were carried out with standard nontoxic vaccines such as Centanit for carcinoma, Sarkogen for sarcoma, and Lymphogran for Hodgkin's disease.

General immunotherapy is used to bolster the patient's overall immunity and to destroy the "tumor milieu" that makes it possible for the cancer to sustain itself and grow. Autovaccines are prepared from extracts from the patient's own teeth and tonsils as well as other nontoxic vaccines designed to boost general resistance to disease.

Ozone therapy, although not a direct aid to the immune system, is also used as a means of increasing the oxygen supply to the cells and destroying viruses and bacteria in the bloodstream. This method of systematically exposing portions of the patient's blood supply to medically pure ozone is not commonly practiced in the United States, but has been used against blood-borne infectious diseases in Germany for more than thirty years. Dr. Issels found the therapy to be effective in purging the blood of oxidation-resistant pesticides and other toxins.

Finally, hyperpyrexia, homeopathy's long-sanctioned induction of fever, is also used in much the same way as ozone therapy to make life uncomfortable for the tumor. Once a month, patients get a "fever shot," which can raise the body temperature as high as 105°F, where it stays for several minutes while the patient is under constant medical supervision.

While Dr. Issels may not have shared the enthusiasm of the ancient Greek physician who remarked, "Give me a chance to produce fever, and I can cure all illness," he knew that fever was a natural reaction of the body to foreign invaders and that it made these invaders more vulnerable to attack. He also discovered that the number of disease-destroying white blood cells in the patient's bloodstream rose enormously after each fever shot and that the patients uniformly reported feeling much better afterward as their bodies were detoxified. Even localized heating of the tumor area, Dr. Issels discovered, could have effects which, while not as spectacular, were clearly beneficial.

The Results

A landmark study of Dr. Issels's medical records conducted by highly reputed experts confirmed a 16.6 percent cure rate among the terminal patients treated with *Ganzheit* therapy. To understand the significance of this figure, it is necessary to recall that all these patients were terminal, already given up on by conventional medicine. In the United States, for example, such a patient has virtually no chance of survival, let alone of cure.

This distinction between survival and cure is also crucial. For conventional medicine, "cure" simply means that the cancer patient has survived five years after the initial diagnosis. It says nothing about the state of the patient during that time or at its end. Dr. Issels used a different standard.

Dr. Issels continued his fight against cancer throughout his life. In the years before he died in 1998 at the age of ninety, Dr. Issels and colleagues at the Centro Hospitalario Internacional Pacifico, S.A. (CHIPSA) Center for Integrative Medicine refined a program that combined his comprehensive immunotherapy with the similarly holistic approach developed by the late Dr. Max Gerson.

Issels Treatment is currently practiced at a clinic located in Santa Barbara, California, and another in Tijuana, Mexico. The average cost of the standard three-week treatment is $15,000 but can vary depending on the clinic location.

For more information on this therapy, contact:
The Issels Foundation
(888) 447-7357
www.issels.com

The Eclectic Triphasic
Medical System (ETMS)

The Eclectic Triphasic Medical System (ETMS) was pioneered by Donald Yance, a practicing clinical herbalist, certified nutritionist, author of *Dietary, Herbal and Nutritional Strategies for Treating and Preventing Cancer,* and the founder of the Mederi Centre for Natural Healing in Ashland, Oregon. The ETMS approach to cancer incorporates both traditional and modern healing techniques, with an emphasis on herbal medicine. Yance described to me his protocol for treating and preventing cancer:

The foods that I would emphasize in general are first of all the highest quality attainable, as fresh as possible, and organic. I always stress quality and balance. I don't care if you think you should be juicing carrots, beets, and celery; in my opinion they must be organic and they must be fresh. I tend to base a lot of my specifics on the person's health status, the person's genetic makeup, and the type of cancer they have. Of course I am going to emphasize foods that contain a high level of phytochemicals that we know inhibit cancer and possibly can reverse cancer.

Phytochemicals and phytonutrients are new terms that describe plant constituents that are not vitamins or minerals but various compounds that play an important role in cell protection. They protect against the initiation and promotion of cancer. Of the flavones, my favorite is called quercetin, which is found abundantly in broccoli and in onions and is a wonderful inhibitor of a number of different cancer cell lines. Isoflavones are found in the soybean food family. Tryterpines, limolines, and nomlines are found in citrus fruit, mostly in the rind and the oil of the citrus, which can be made into a tea with orange peel, lemon peel, or from the oils. Some of these are in clinical trials for cancer therapy.

Donald Yance describes himself as a big believer in Omega-3 fatty acids. "Not only do they have strong inhibitory effects on cancer growth from many mechanisms, but they also help to feed the body nutrition-wise, particularly combined with protein. I know there are a lot of different viewpoints on this topic. Do I need to build up this person while at the same time detoxifying them? That is where you play the balance between foods that will build a person and inhibit cancer, and foods that will detoxify the person."

So, a combination of detoxification and a health-restoring diet is essential to the Yance approach.

Detoxification

Yance's detoxifying program includes using Epsom salt baths to raise the body temperature. As he notes, "Most people with cancer have a very subnormal body temperature. It is important to get the body's immune system activated by raising the body temperature. When people are in contact with some sort of pathogen, the body's natural response is to secrete pyrogens that raise the body's temperature. We do this artificially because cancer does not provoke the usual immunological reaction, so we do things to help that." He mixes essential oils, mostly lavender, into the bathtub and gives patients an herbal compound along with an herbal tea.

Another measure focuses on liver detoxifying, which relies on a number of different plant compounds along with various supplements. "I favor alpha-lipoic acid combined with some very concentrated forms of herbs, particularly turmeric. Alpha-lipoic acid is a highly absorbable nutrient that is both fat- and water-soluble. In my opinion it is the first precursor of glutathione, which is part of the phase II liver enzyme detoxifying system. It helps detoxify xenoestrogens, lipid-soluble toxins, some other drugs and pollutants, and possibly some other things like dead cancer cells. The liver is the main vehicle for breaking these things down and helping the body secrete them. The dosage I use is 300 mg of lipoic acid twice per day." In addition, he uses a compound of standardized curcuminoids, the active constituent in turmeric. One gram is administered three or four times per day on an empty stomach combined with bromelain, an enzyme from pineapple that interacts with the turmeric and with quercetin. The dosages of quercetin and bromelain are the same, one gram three or four times per day on an empty stomach. According to Yance, these three compounds have a synergistic effect in that they all help each other be absorbed more efficiently.

Other Herbs

Yance believes several other common herbs can benefit cancer patients. "An interesting plant that I use quite a bit in breast cancer is an herb called pulsatilla, which has no anticancer activity but tends to lift a person's spirit. I think that ability is the first and foremost part of any person's treatment." Schisandra, known as a five-spice herb in Chinese medicine because it has salt, sweet, bitter, pungent, and sour taste all in one plant, "is a wonderful hepatic protective agent and detoxifier and also is used to treat nervous exhaustion. It helps the body's endocrine system with the stress of having cancer. It balances the pH of the digestive system, which may be too alkaline or too acidic, and so improves the ability of the body to absorb. It is perhaps the most powerful liver protective agent of all plants." Red clover is effective with some of the hormonal type cancers, like breast cancer and prostate cancer. "Because of the isoflavones and curcuminoids present in this plant, I use a 1:1 extract of red clover instead of the over-the-counter preparations of 1:5, which are not as strong. I make a decoction (a tea you prepare by boiling until the water is two-thirds evaporated and then straining before consumption) of blossoms of red clover, which is also very nice."

Licorice is also used in herbal treatments. "It has hormone-regulating properties and liver-protective properties; it is a demulcent, so it soothes mucus membranes; and it is a precursor to aldosterone. Aldosterone is the hormone that tells the body to hold onto fluids. If a person has very dry skin, and every time they drink liquid, they urinate it right out of their bodies, their blood pressure tends to be very low; they may have low levels of aldosterone, so think of using a little licorice."

Emotional and Spiritual Health

Attitude, love, and spirituality play a part in healing cancer, as in many other diseases. Donald Yance believes attending to a patient's emotional and spiritual health is the essence of healing. Reducing a patient's fear of cancer is important. Fear interferes with sleep, which is essential for detoxification as the body does most of its detoxifying while in the deepest rest.

"Fear is an obstacle in the way of healing, and I believe this is where you tap into a person's spirit. Once a person is comfortable with who they are spiritually, they no longer have fear. The whole body, mind, and spirit are interrelated. When you feel comfortable with who you are spiritually you don't worry about things as much."

Yance works with patients to come to terms with the inevitability of eventual death. "I always explain that we are all going to ultimately die. We need to come to grips with that and not fixate on it. Let's think about the living, let's think about today, let's think about how we can step forward and be healed, because you don't want to live miserably anyway. Let's think about how you can enrich yourself on all levels and that everything complements each other. One of my great loves for plant medicine is that plants are here on earth just like we are, and they exude a tremendous amount of healing."

Treatment Details

The typical cost of ETMS cancer treatment administered by Donald Yance and his colleagues at the Mederi Centre for Natural Healing in Ashland, Oregon, is $1,000 per month.

For more information on this therapy, contact:
Mederi Centre for Natural Healing
(541) 488-3133
www.mederifoundation.org

Antineoplaston Therapy

Nearly 50 years ago, a medical student in Poland took a new and different approach to cancer research. He decided to find out why all people don't have cancer. Everyone is exposed to the same known and unknown causative agents of this disease. What is different about the people who never contract it? Is this difference the key to developing a cure?

The Discovery: Dr. Stanislaw Burzynski

Dr. Stanislaw Burzynski believes so. Now working out of a research facility he founded in 1977 in Houston, Texas, Dr. Burzynski has successfully treated about 2,000 patients with advanced cancer. Most of these people turned to him as a last resort when conventional treatment with radiation, chemotherapy, and surgery had failed. What they found was a therapy based not on the abuse of the body's built-in defense systems but rather on the transformation of cancerous cells into healthy, normal tissue.

Dr. Burzynski's solution lies in a group of chemical substances, part of a larger group of chemical compounds called peptides, that exist in every human body. His research points to a severe shortage of these substances—called antineoplastons—in cancer patients. Simply stated, antineoplastons are a special class of peptides, found in the body, that combat neoplastons—abnormal cells or cancer cells. Antineoplastons could be the vehicle needed by the body to ward off and even reverse the development of these cancerous cells. Dr. Burzynski has put this theory into action, treating patients by reintroducing antineoplastons into the bloodstream, either intravenously or orally with capsules. In many cases, tumors shrank in size or actually disappeared. Some patients even experienced complete remission of their cancers, and years of follow-up study have revealed no sign of any return.

Such results are almost unbelievable. Dr. Burzynski appears to have tapped the power of antineoplastons to naturally "reprogram" cancer cells. His approach could virtually eliminate the need to destroy these cells or remove the tumors they create. This therapy was not developed overnight. It took Dr. Burzynski nearly three decades of research, first in Poland, then at the Baylor College of Medicine in Houston, Texas, and ultimately at the Burzynski Research Institute in Houston. During this time, Dr. Burzynski zeroed in on the substance he named "antineoplaston." But to get back to Dr. Burzynski's original concern, why do tumors develop in the first place?

Why Tumors Develop

According to Burzynski's theory, cancer is caused primarily by an information-processing error. Good information produces healthy cells; bad information results in cancerous cells. Antineoplastons are important because they carry "good" information to the cells. They can "tell" the cells to develop normally.

All cells start out with specific goals. Some turn into skin, some into blood vessels, some into bone or other body tissues. However, they will never go on to perform these highly specialized functions in the body unless they go through a process called *differentiation*. Cancer cells, or neoplastons, which everybody produces regularly, never differentiate. They are abnormal cells that the healthy body rejects and destroys because they have not received good information and therefore have no constructive role to play. When the body is in a weakened state, these neoplastons are not destroyed but rather are left at the mercy of cancer-causing agents that invade the system and "turn them on." They begin to multiply, forming large, constantly growing lumps. They are victims of bad information and assume a destructive role in the body.

This is where antineoplastons come in—as a means of relaying positive messages. Antineoplastons are able to send instructions to abnormal or cancerous cells that can then allow them to differentiate or specialize, thus restoring the body's normal defense mechanisms. The beauty of the treatment is that harmful drugs, radiation, and surgery are not required. The body virtually heals itself.

A Biochemical Defense System

According to the research done by Dr. Burzynski and others in the United States as well as abroad, antineoplastons are components of a biochemical defense system that parallels our immune system. Unlike the immune system, which protects us by destroying invading agents or defective cells, this biochemical defense system protects us by reprogramming, or normalizing, defective cells. Errors in cell programming may lead to such diverse disorders as cancer, benign tumors, certain skin diseases, AIDS, and Parkinson's disease.

Evolution of a Therapy

Stanislaw Burzynski was born into a family with a passion for learning. His parents had university degrees, his father a total of five before retiring as a university professor. Stanislaw followed suit, becoming at age twenty-five one of Poland's youngest men ever to earn both an MD and a PhD. He began his research at one of Poland's finest medical schools, the Lublin Medical Academy. Its prestigious faculty provided the mentors he needed to shape his embryonic theories on anticancer defense mechanisms.

The Polish government eventually allowed him to emigrate to the United States, and by 1970 Dr. Burzynski had become a staff member at Baylor College of Medicine, continuing his theories about the causes and treatments of cancer. Because his research had been interrupted by obligatory military service, nearly a decade had passed since he had fixed on the notion that the human body must possess a built-in system to resist cancer and similar diseases. He believed that without this system, no one could hope to ward off the cancer-creating "sea of carcinogens" that surround us. Of course, believing that a natural defense system exists does not explain what it is made up of and how it works, but mentors from his university days offered some clues.

From a former chemistry professor Dr. Burzynski had learned about the information-carrying peptides, which are related to the antineoplastons he had yet to uncover. Other clues had come from Dr. Marian Mazur, professor at the Polish Academy of Science and a widely acclaimed authority in the cybernetic field of science. Cybernetics looks at how systems work; one of its key elements is feedback, which provides a way to control and communicate within a system. If cancer cells become destructive because they have received only bad information, the task is not to kill them but to get the right information to them to make them normal and healthy. Cybernetics provides insight into the nature of improving communications within a system so that the desired information or feedback is properly transmitted. A household thermostat is an example of a feedback device: a tool used to close the gap between an actual result—say, room temperature of 90 degrees—and a desired result—a more comfortable 70 degrees.

Dr. Burzynski concluded that the active ingredient of the body's cancer defense system might be found in the family of peptides—small blood proteins—which are known to communicate with and affect the growth of cells. Within that system, these substances could operate as a feedback device to correct the difference between actual cancer cells and the desired healthy cells, or to reprogram cancer cells with good information so that they could become constructive and vital instead of pathogenic.

Peptides are a popular subject of modern medical research. Nearly fifty different types have been found that can stimulate cell growth. One, known as peptide T, is attracting attention for its potential in treating AIDS. Dr. Burzynski is thus by no means the only scientist exploring the potency of peptides, but he has been at it longer than most and has achieved findings unique to cancer therapy.

An early discovery involved the level of peptides in advanced cancer patients. Their blood samples revealed only 2–3 percent of the amount typically found in healthy bodies—a drastic difference. If peptides, as Dr. Burzynski assumed, played a role in the body's natural defense system, these cancer patients had at some point been disarmed. They were victims of misinformation, because there were not enough peptides to carry good information to the cancer cells.

The next task was to determine exactly what kind of peptides cancerous bodies lack. Burzynski put his doctorate in biochemistry to good use, studying the makeup and structure of the deficient substances and uncovering an interesting effect. When applied to tissue cultures, the peptides missing from cancer patients actually suppressed the growth of human cancer cells.

But while progress was evident, the puzzle was far from solved. It was not enough to know that antineoplastons could carry appropriate information to cancerous cells; it had to be determined how to get them to do it in order to ameliorate tumor growths. Dr. Burzynski turned to his knowledge of systems, cybernetic science, and information theory. The idea of using feedback to adjust and correct an obvious imbalance seemed appropriate to the possible role of antineoplastons in treating cancer.

The Treatment: Reprogramming Cancer Cells

Dr. Burzynski's concept constituted a scientific leap, yet it appears amazingly simple in light of the most basic function peptides perform: they transmit information to the cells. Some aim to spur on, others to inhibit, cellular growth, but they all do it by sending messages the body can obey.

Dr. Burzynski likens the process to the use of the alphabet: "It's like having twenty-six alphabet letters—you can create an infinite variety of words."[356] Using the right "code" becomes the key to reprogramming cancerous cells. Theoretically, it is possible to stop a peptide messenger carrying dangerous, damaging goods and hand over a more beneficent, favorable package for it to deliver instead.

The best time to change the peptide code is when cells are new and immature. Guided by good information, the cells can successfully pass through all the normal stages of development. They can gradually take on the special traits they need to serve different parts of the body—in other words, differentiate. When cells differentiate, they have reached maturity. Imagine being stuck in childhood or puberty, never given the means to change and grow into a fully functioning adult. This is the state of a cancer cell. It doesn't know how to differentiate and mature, because its genetic code is garbled. In a healthy body with a sufficient level of peptides and antineoplastons, good information is quickly communicated to the cancer cell, and the cell is rendered harmless. But when these peptide levels are low, the cancer cell continues to be victimized by the wrong information. Dr. Burzynski's treatment is aimed at ending the cancer cell's confusion. He puts antineoplastons into the bloodstream to carry the proper genetic code, halt the growth of useless tumors, and encourage cancer cells to differentiate.

Antineoplastons are not foreign substances. Because they appear naturally in the body—and evidently are found at a much higher level in healthy bodies—they don't pose a toxic threat. This fact alone sets Dr. Burzynski's approach miles apart from traditional cancer therapies. Radiation treatments and chemotherapy destroy cancer cells but also destroy any other cells in their path.

Two significant observations have been made about the side effects of antineoplaston treatment. First, most patients experience virtually no side effects. The few that have appeared have been minor, short-lived, and easily controlled, such as skin rashes, chills, and fever. The second and more remarkable observation is that the treatment can actually create positive side effects in decided contrast to traditional medical treatments. Patients have shown increases in white and red blood cell counts, decreases in blood cholesterol, and stimulated skin growth; these and other effects are known to aid the body's natural healing powers. Antineoplaston therapy has tremendous promise not just in theory but in practice.

However, a new medicine or medical treatment is not accepted overnight. The medical and scientific communities as well as certain governmental bodies set rigid testing standards to ensure the safety and effectiveness of every supposed curative. Antineoplastons are no exception.

Tests and Results

For several decades, Dr. Burzynski has been subjecting his theory to the testing procedure required to prove its worth, and it is holding up well under pressure. More than 60 percent of the patients treated during the Burzynski Research Institute's phase I testing showed considerable improvement.

Each phase of testing has different goals. Phase I is designed to examine any side effects that may occur and to determine proper dosages of the antineoplaston "medicine." Phase II entails a more specific study of whether and how the medicine acts to reduce or eliminate cancerous growth, and phase III takes an even closer look at these issues, among larger groups of people with the same types of cancer.

When phase I clinical trials began, Dr. Burzynski didn't expect much in the way of an anticancer effect. His aim was to find out how much medicine patients should be given, starting with very small doses that could be increased over time. He had no way of knowing but could only suspect which kinds of cancer would respond best to his treatment. What he expected and what he got were two different things.

The results in the best cases of twenty different phase I trials showed significant anticancer activity. In the most successful trial, not only did more than 60 percent of the patients respond to treatment; more than 20 percent remained cancer-free for over five years. These patients suffered from some of the most serious and difficult-to-treat forms of cancer, including advanced lung and bladder cancer, and malignant mesothelioma—a type of cancer that results from asbestos exposure and is especially resistant to traditional medicine.

In phase II trials, patients are grouped according to their basic type of cancer. Depending on how and where those basic types develop in the body, different phase II treatments are tried. For example, in current trials with breast cancer, treatment varies depending on whether the disease has spread to the lungs or to the liver or bones.

In 1992, twenty-four patients with malignant lymphoma (cancer of the lymphatic system) had been treated in phase II trials. Chemotherapy had failed to help nearly 70 percent of these patients. Only certain forms of this cancer, such as Hodgkin's disease, have ever shown real success from conventional treatment. But with antineoplaston care, 85 percent showed significant improvement.

The most impressive results have been in brain cancers (astrocytoma stages III and IV, and glioblastoma) and metastatic cancer of the prostate. In a small phase II trial of astrocytoma conducted by Dr. Burzynski, twenty patients were enrolled. All diagnoses were confirmed by biopsy. All but one patient had received (and failed) one or more prior standard therapies. Of the twenty patients Dr. Burzynski treated, four achieved complete remission and two others partial remission. The responses of ten patients were classified as objective stabilization (less than 50 percent decrease of tumor size). Since the end of this study in May 1990, some of these patients have achieved partial and even complete remission.

In another phase II study of fourteen patients with stage IV prostate cancer resistant to hormonal treatment, two complete and three partial remissions were reported, while seven patients obtained objective stabilization.

In a 1997 interview, Dr. Burzynski offered more of the clinic's success stories:

When we started our program, we concentrated on the type of cancers that are uniformly deadly, such terrible types of malignant tumors as primary malignant brain tumors that are known in medical terminology as astrocytoma, glioblastoma, and medulla blastoma. Practically everybody who develops high-grade astrocytoma or glioblastoma dies from the disease. There's no cure available, and the death comes quickly, usually within a year.

We concentrated on the treatment of such highly malignant tumors to prove a point that antineoplastons work. Otherwise, if there are some other treatments available, we could be accused of perhaps using these additional treatments which could make the tumors disappear. But those treatments do not exist. If we are able to eliminate highly malignant brain tumors by the use of antineoplastons, these are the first cases in medical history of this happening. Because we concentrate our efforts on the treatment of such bad malignant brain tumors, of course, most of our statistics concentrate on these tumors. We already finished three clinical trials, phase II trials, in such malignant brain tumors. And we found that the success rate of the patients who are responding to the treatment is between 67 to 80 percent among these trials, which means that only 20 percent to 33 percent of the patients do not have any proper response to the treatment.

We already have long-term follow-up for some of these patients, including an eight-year follow-up when the tumors disappeared and did not come back. We can say that we were able to not only decrease and eliminate these tumors, but also cure a number of patients from these tumors. We continue to have clinical trials in different types of malignant brain tumors. Currently, we have over twenty different clinical trials in the area of malignant brain tumors, and we are accepting the patients through such trials. If somebody is interested we can, of course, offer him the treatment, and then he can go back home and continue the treatment under the care of his doctor.[357]

The Clinic

The Burzynski Clinic in southwest Houston currently sees approximately 70–120 patients each month. The clinic operates on an outpatient basis. The average period of care involves an intensive two- to three-week period with patients visiting the clinic daily followed by an additional four to twelve months of self-administered care at home. The average cost of treatment is between $25,000 and $30,000.

The antineoplastons that have been responsible for the dramatic results mentioned above are manufactured in Dr. Burzynski's plant in Stafford, Texas. According to Dr. Burzynski, they are considered a form of chemotherapy because a chemotherapeutic agent is technically any mixture of chemicals that combat cancer. However, they do not have the devastating side effects of the traditional class of chemotherapeutic drugs because they are formulations that are identical to proteins that are present in the body. Natural antineoplastons are small proteins isolated from human urine or blood. Synthetic antineoplastons are chemically identical to the natural proteins but are synthetically derived. Synthetics are easier and cheaper to manufacture and are even more efficacious in treating specific cancers such as brain and prostate cancer. Other cancers, though, respond better to the natural substances.

Dr. Burzynski uses a deliberately coordinated assortment of antineoplastons, both synthetic and natural, as the case requires. When he thinks it is appropriate, he refers patients for other types of treatment (chemotherapy, radiation, or surgery) to augment the antineoplaston injection or capsule therapy. While he has had little success with cancer of the testicles and childhood leukemia, he has had astounding results with brain tumors, malignant lymphomas, and cancer of the bladder and prostate.

The Burzynski clinic's report from January 2012 shows that out of 1,849 patients treated for the fifteen most common cancer types treated at the clinic, the average objective response (percentage of individuals whose cancer has measurably improved) was at 50 percent. For some cancers, including ovarian and non-Hodgkin's lymphoma, the objective response exceeded 60 percent. In all but three of the fifteen most commonly treated cancers, a greater percentage of patients experienced stable disease (where the condition is not decreasing or increasing in extent or severity) rather than progressive disease (where the condition worsens).

Looking to the Future

There are currently ten FDA-sponsored clinical trials underway to assess the antineoplaston treatment in treating patients with various forms of cancer. As of January 2012, there is one open clinical trial.

The possibilities of Dr. Burzynski's therapy appear endless. Antineoplastons correct (i.e., stop) cancer development in a way the body understands and easily tolerates. Even with phase I treatments, which aren't intended to produce maximum benefits, some patients emerged cancer-free. Of course, successful outcomes result from traditional approaches as well. Careful surgery can aid recovery, and chemotherapy has had particular success with rarer types of cancer such as Hodgkin's disease and childhood leukemia.

What Dr. Burzynski offers is an opportunity to use and strengthen the body's natural defense system. The need to explore and develop antineoplastons and other safe remedies will continue as long as people are exposed to air pollution, radiation, chemicals, ultraviolet rays, and other carcinogenic toxins.

For more information on this therapy, contact:
Burzynski Clinic
9432 Katy Freeway
Houston, TX 77055
(800) 714-7181
www.burzynskiclinic.com

Dr. Burzynski and his colleagues routinely publish the results of their latest research at www.burzynskiclinic.com/publications .html.

Testimonials

Theresa on Stage IV Lymphoma: In 1984, after the birth of my daughter, I had a biopsy that showed that I had stage IV lymphoma. My doctors said that I should go on chemotherapy right away, even though I wouldn't be able to get rid of the lymphoma. They said it was incurable.

I had a second opinion and they said the same thing, but they said they could check it for a while and not give me any chemo right away. I never did end up having chemotherapy or radiation.

Today, I'm great, thanks to Dr. Burzynski. He gave me the antineoplaston therapy, which means anticancer. It's a peptide that he discovered. Apparently, most peptides are growth-enhancing peptides. Peptides are precursors to amino acids, which are the precursors to proteins. The peptides that he found are peptides that inhibit the growth of certain types of cells. Rather than killing the cancer cells along with a lot of other healthy cells, peptides just keep the cancer cells from growing. They live out their lifespan, and then they die off. Eventually, whatever organ is affected is turned back into a healthy organ. That's what happened with me.

While I was healing, I made a lot of changes. I realized I had a lot of anger that I wasn't dealing with. I was taught that anger is bad and hurtful, and I developed a way of suppressing my anger while not even knowing that I had it. So one part of getting well, a big part, was coming more to terms with my anger, accepting it, and expressing it appropriately, rather than stuffing it inside and turning it into cancer.

Another aspect was learning to visualize my cancer going away, and holding a more positive view of my future. I did change a lot of things. I changed my job, and I changed a lot of my relationships. I went through a lot of changes.

Today, I feel a lot different than I did then. I'm much more aware of my feelings, and physically I feel a lot better. Over the months that I worked with Dr. Burzynski's medicine, I saw my cancer gradually disappear. I was grateful to be able to deal with my healing process in a nontoxic way, and I'm really grateful to be alive.

Ellen on Intestinal Asbestos Cancer: This is the same type of cancer that Steve McQueen died of. It was a slow-growing cancer. I was on 250 pain pills a month for ten years. Finally, Sloan-Kettering gave me two years to live. I called Dr. Burzynski and asked him if he could help me. After the first week of treatment, I was off the pain pills. I had no side effects. I was on his program for nine months, and I got cured.

Tessie on Lymphoma: I was advised to get chemotherapy, which I started in June 1992. In July 1993, it reappeared in my neck. My doctor said that with my condition, chemotherapy might help. But the second time that I started chemotherapy, the tumor was not getting smaller.

I had the feeling that I had to do something different. I decided to go to Dr. Burzynski because I got tired of the chemotherapy. I told my doctor that I was going to stop the chemotherapy and get a second opinion. My doctor was shocked, and he started putting pressure on me to go back on chemotherapy. He said I would lose ground, but I didn't. Today, I am free of cancer.

Actually, the chemotherapy was causing me to lose ground. I was so weak from it that I was running a fever. I had bronchitis, and I had pneumonia. My heart was also damaged from the chemotherapy. After getting well, I went back to my doctor for blood tests to send to Dr. Burzynski.

Mary Jo on Low-Grade Non-Hodgkin's Lymphoma, Stage IV: I was told that I needed a bone marrow transplant, massive chemotherapy, total body irradiation, and six weeks of total isolation in a hospital. My doctor gave me no guarantee, but he said that this was my only chance for a cure. My other option was to take chemotherapy and radiation every two years. I already had a tumor on the side of my neck, which was growing. If I didn't follow his advice, he said it would press against my organs and I would die.

I did some more research. That's when I heard about Dr. Burzynski's totally nontoxic treatment. I thought I would be foolish not to try it. When I called my doctor at UCLA, he was adamant that I not start Dr. Burzynski's treatment, but I did it anyway.

My medical records are open to everybody. Every CT scan I had showed a reduction. I have maintained my doctor at UCLA who says, over and over again, "I can't say it's not working, but I don't know why it's working." He calls me a spontaneous remission.

One thing that is so important about Dr. Burzynski's treatment is that it is totally nontoxic. I lived a completely normal life while I was on it. I was able to do grocery shopping, drive my kids' car pools, everything.

Revici Therapy

The late biochemist and physician Dr. Emmanuel Revici was the innovator of a remarkable nontoxic form of chemotherapy that has effectively treated different forms of cancer and other illnesses. During the first part of his long career, which began in the 1920s, Dr. Revici conducted groundbreaking research into the role of lipids, which are fundamental building blocks of human biology, in the development of cancer. Much of Dr. Revici's studies centered on the observation that lipids are insoluble in blood and therefore selectively absorbed by damaged body tissue. His research also determined that tumors have a high concentration of abnormal free lipids.

Using this information, Dr. Revici devised a method in which natural substances derived from plant, mineral, and animal material could be integrated with lipids to create a special compound. By introducing these compounds to the bloodstream, the treatment transports therapeutic agents to diseased and abnormal tissue where they help restore normal body function. In treating cancer patients, Revici used selenium compounds due to their exceptional capacity to be absorbed by tumors and subsequently destroy cancer cells and shrink the size of tumors.

Treatment Success
Revici Medical, the New York–based nonprofit organization dedicated to advancing the work of Dr. Revici, reports that the organization has compiled numerous case studies that detail

significant improvement in the condition of patients with prostate, kidney, breast, pancreatic, and other cancers. In some cases, a full clinical remission has been reported. Because the substances added to these lipid compounds are natural and nontoxic, the majority of patients taking Revici's medications experience no significant adverse reactions.

Raphael Kellman, MD, practices an integrative cancer treatment that incorporates the principles of the Revici Therapy. The therapy aims to improve the function of cell, organ, and systems through natural medicine and technologies designed to improve oxygenation and restore homeostasis.

For more information on this therapy, contact:
Raphael Kellman, MD
150 East 55th Street, 6th Floor
New York, NY 10022
(212) 717-1118
raphaelkellmanmd.com

Testimonials

Fernando on Prostate Cancer: I was diagnosed for prostate cancer at age fifty-six. I scored 8 on the Gleason scale, which I understand is rather high. The cells were highly undifferentiated, which I understand makes them proliferate more rapidly. And I was also at a relatively young age to get prostate cancer. Those three things, everyone seemed to agree, would make it more aggressive. My urologist immediately suggested a radical prostatectomy. I declined, for two reasons, because I was not and am not convinced that invasive therapies lengthen the lifespan, and on the other hand, they do alter your lifestyle tremendously, and I was not ready to undergo the changes that operations of that sort apparently cause you. After some research, I decided to come to Dr. Revici, and I'm very happy that I did.

I've also made changes to my lifestyle, nutritionally and with supplementation. I've started to take ozone therapy. Basically, what Dr. Revici's therapy did to an extremely aggressive carcinoma is apparently to have stopped it in its tracks. From what I've heard from mainstream doctors and urologists . . . the way it seemed from the outset was that I did not have much time—two and a half or three years. Here I am, with lots of energy and very enthusiastic about the response my body has had to Dr. Revici's therapy. I've been in remission five years, and I hope we can extend that indefinitely.

Robert on Angiosarcoma: I discovered that I had a lump in my jaw. I went through a series of extensive tests, including two biopsies, one in the hospital and one outside. It included MRIs, CT scans, X-rays, and that sort of thing. Out of that came the diagnosis of angiosarcoma. Basically, the doctor who was associated with Georgetown Hospital told me that with this diagnosis I had about one chance in ten of being alive in five years. He said that that particular kind of cancer was not treatable by any of the usual techniques, namely surgery, radiation, or chemotherapy.

Given that kind of prognosis, and given the lack of treatment options, I decided it was time to look elsewhere for treatment. My wife had worked with a lady who was a former patient of Dr. Revici, so I knew of Dr. Revici through her and contacted the doctor. I was actively under his care for about six years. By that I mean I went to see him in his office approximately once a month. The treatment consisted primarily of capsules that I took orally. He put me on a number of different medications.

What struck me about his treatment is that he tailors it to the person. He would sometimes have me on two or three medications. He would tell me to call him in three or four days, and he might change the medication, depending upon how I was reacting to it. Over that period, he probably had me on a couple dozen different things. I have not been receiving treatment for a little over a year.

His office asked me to have an MRI done, which I did, and a couple of months ago, I sent them the results. Basically, the MRI shows that in the last three years, there has been no growth at all in the tumor.

Ozone Therapy

Not to be confused with atmospheric ozone, medical ozone is pure and concentrated, and has unique healing properties. Although ozone therapy is not widely practiced in the United States, Europeans and Cubans have been benefiting from these treatments for years.

Ozone is used both prophylactically and as a treatment for a wide variety of diseases, including cancer. An antineoplastic substance (one that inhibits the growth of tumors), ozone stimulates the production of white blood cells and increases production of alpha interferon, interleukin-2, and tumor necrosis factor (a protein that can kill tumor cells). It has also been found to enhance the action of various antitumor drugs.

According to the naturopathic physician Dr. Stanley Beyerle, prostate cancer patients often respond quite well to ozone treatment if the cancer is left encapsulated (that is, not biopsied). Other types of cancer that Beyerle has treated effectively using ozone therapy are tonsillar, throat, ovarian, colon, and breast cancer.[358]

Medical ozone is delivered in various ways. One way is to mix a portion of the patient's blood, outside the body, with a dose of ozone/oxygen, and then reintroduce the blood into the circulation. Another is for the ozone to be introduced into the rectum; a third is for the patient to drink ozonated water.

Testimonials

Richard on Prostate Cancer: Before discovering that I had prostate cancer, I had severe pains, especially during sexual relations. I was passing blood and had an awful time urinating. I went to see a specialist. After taking tests, he told me I had a solid cancer and that he needed to operate.

Fortunately, I learned through someone else about a doctor in Mexico. When I got to the clinic, my prostate count was 78. I began ozone treatments, and after three weeks, my count was down to 37. I continued treatments at home, and after six months, my count was down to zero. I continue using ozone to this very day. I take it in different ways. I have an ozone machine, and I use it when taking a bath, and I ozonate my drinking water as well. I use it a lot, because I feel if I don't, the cancer will come back.

Since my treatments, I feel better than I have felt in years. Now I can pass water without a problem. I can work and feel very good. I am more than pleased.

If it hadn't been for the ozone treatments, I wouldn't be here today, because that cancer would have had me. Surgery would have done no good.

Angelo on Colorectal Cancer with Metastases to the Liver: I was feeling tired every day and coming home to take a nap in the afternoon. That wasn't me. I had been a real active person all my life. My wife suggested that I take a blood test to see if anything was wrong. I did, and my doctor found that my blood was low. He suggested that I wait another week before taking another test, which I did. My blood was still low, so he suggested a colonoscopy. I went and had it done. The colonoscopy found a tumor in my colon. I had it operated on and taken out. The surgeon told me that he successfully removed it and that there was no more cancer there.

About three months later, I had a CT scan done that found spots on my liver. The cancer had metastasized on my liver. I received chemotherapy treatments for approximately six months. After the first set of treatments, another test was taken, which found that chemotherapy hadn't done any good. I continued with the chemotherapy for another three months. When that didn't help, the doctor said that there was nothing more he could do for me. I asked if I should continue with the chemo or just sit and die. He shrugged his shoulders, as if to say there was nothing more he could do for me. I asked the doctor how much time he thought I had and he said three to four months.

My son, who was there with me, had heard about a holistic program at Santa Monica Hospital utilizing ozone and vitamin therapy. He said I should take the treatments there, and I did. I received treatments for twenty-one days. They asked me to wait for eight weeks before having a CT scan. When I finally took the CT scan, the radiologist called my doctor and told him that he had never read a CT scan like mine before. It showed that the cancer cells in my liver had become capsulized. That prevented them from spreading.

The cancer cells have remained encapsulated, and I've been in remission for a year and a half. There is no question about it. The ozone treatment saved my life. In fact, I have so much faith in it now that I plan on going there every year and a half just to make sure that it stays that way.

Jane on Breast Cancer: I was diagnosed in 1989 with breast cancer, for which I had a modified radical mastectomy. I had numerous surgeries before that time as well. I wasn't really having any life at that point in time. I was a sick person waiting to die. They had cut out some of the cancer, but I wasn't well. A friend of mine finally advised me not to have any more of those treatments because they were killing me.

I had the book *Third Opinion,* which had something in it about Dr. Donsbach. I called Santa Monica Hospital and went down there. I was astounded by the humaneness of the Santa Monica Hospital. In other hospitals, I had some negative experiences where I felt totally robbed of all dignity and where I was treated like a specimen.

Santa Monica had a program that I could tolerate. I had decided that I was not going to have any more cutting, any more radiation, or any more chemo. There would be no more invasive procedures.

The first week I felt really, really sick because I was detoxifying from all the chemicals in my system. I had been on ten different medications for multiple problems. Besides cancer, I had ulcers, asthma, everything you could possibly imagine. The cancer had set off a systems reaction, and I was having problems in every part of my body.

After about the tenth day, I started to feel like getting out of bed. I began to participate in the therapies and started beach walks. I continued to get better and better.

I have been there six or seven times because I had some tumors in the other breast as well. I received ozone, hyperthermia, and thymus injections.

I don't have any tumors now. Most of all, I have a life. I work full-time, and I play an active role in the lives of my granddaughter and daughters. I am able to go to church. I participate in library programs. I walk on the beach every day. I follow my program.

I learned things in the hospital that I need to be real careful with. Santa Monica Hospital will be the first place I go to if I begin developing symptoms. I don't think I will, though. I think I'm cured.

Vaccines

When some of a patient's own cancer cells are combined in a laboratory with some of his or her white blood cells, it's possible—in some cases—to create a personalized vaccine that works to stimulate the patient's immune system to destroy the cancer. One such vaccine approach to cancer comes from Dr. William Coley, who practiced in the early part of the twentieth century. He found that certain inactivated bacteria could be given to patients to energize their immune systems against cancer. It was as if, by first fighting against the weaker opponent, the bacteria, the body built up its defenses and became more able to fight the cancer. Research has shown this treatment to be of significant value, although a perceived drawback is the fever that develops shortly after the vaccine is given. This, according to proponents of Coley's treatment, is actually a sign that the vaccine is working, and should not be suppressed.[359]

Testimonials

Harry on Massive Tumor outside Colon: I was given six months to a year to live. The surgeon said for me to live it up, and eat and do anything I wanted to do. He sent me to the oncologist, who told me that they could give me treatments but that I had about a 15 percent chance of being helped, and even if I was helped, the treatments would only increase my longevity by a couple of months. I was discouraged with that, so I made some trips to Mexico to study various alternative treatment approaches. Then I got a newsletter from a friend of mine about 714-X and I decided to try it because it was something I felt I could continue on.

My son gave me the injections, which were painless. We followed this program for six months. The total program consisted of 168 shots. Right after I started taking the 714-X, I felt better. I feel just fine now.

When I started on this program, my son turned my way of living around 180 degrees. He prepared an organic diet for me. I cut out alcohol and cut down on cigar smoking to one in the morning and one at night.

Since then, I have felt much better than I have in years. The 714-X stimulated my immune system back to normal.

I went back to my doctor two years later and was given a colonoscopy and some other tests. Tests showed that the tumor had not enlarged and that the growth had stopped. It became dormant. The oncologist wanted to see me, I guess, out of curiosity. He told me that I have a 60 percent better chance of survival. He said that, eventually, the tumor will shrink and then disappear.

Rick on Leukemia: At first, I tried chemotherapy, but it failed to work five times. After each treatment, I would experience a relapse because my leukemia was so aggressive. I was working on my next option, a bone marrow transplant. Iowa City had a few matches for me. The first one they tested was almost a perfect match, so I went in and had the transplant done. They gave me a 5 percent chance of actually making it through the transplant. Even if I made it through the transplant, I only had another 5 percent chance of cure. I survived the transplant but, three months later, my blood tests were really bad. My platelets never did recover completely.

I continued looking for answers. I had a live cell blood analysis done, which tells you more than a CBC [complete blood count] or any test given in conventional medicine. According to my test, it was obvious that I was relapsing from the transplant. My relapse wasn't documented by conventional medicine, but, of course, they don't use this method, so it doesn't matter. I knew, and other people knew.

Eventually, I went back on alternative therapies. Three weeks after getting back on the 714-X, my blood counts, every single one of them, returned to within the normal range. It was amazing. Everybody was astounded by it. I don't know what to attribute it to, but I do know that something helped me. I had my transplant in January 1994. I recovered around April, and here it is May 1995. I've had normal blood tests ever since.

Gary Null's Healthy and Delicious Anticancer Recipes

The following recipes coincide with my recommendations for healthy eating—namely, these meals aim to include those foods which actively fight cancer, and exclude those foods which have been shown to be carcinogenic.

Appetizers

BARLEY WITH COLLARD GREENS AND LEEKS
1 cup collard greens, sliced thin
¼ cup vegetable broth
½ cup leeks, sliced
2 cloves garlic, minced
1 cup fresh tomatoes, chopped
¾ cup mushrooms, sliced (reserve a few slices for garnish)
½ cup red bell peppers, sliced
¼ cup fresh parsley, chopped

½ teaspoon dried oregano
Sea salt to taste
½ teaspoon freshly ground black pepper
3 cups barley, cooked

Place the collard greens in a steamer and steam over boiling water for 20 minutes.

Heat the vegetable broth in a skillet and sauté the leeks and garlic for about 3 minutes until tender.

Add the tomatoes, mushrooms, bell pepper, parsley, oregano, salt, and black pepper, and sauté for about 10 minutes, stirring frequently.

Add the steamed collard greens and sauté for an additional 5 minutes.

Garnish with sliced mushrooms and serve with cooked barley.

Yield: 2 servings

BAVARIAN CABBAGE

¼ cup vegetable broth
1 small yellow onion, diced
1 clove garlic, chopped
1 ounce kombu or arame seaweed, soaked in water for about
    10 minutes to reconstitute
1 cup green cabbage, shredded
½ cup red cabbage, shredded
1 Granny Smith apple, diced
1 teaspoon maple syrup
Sea salt to taste
½ teaspoon freshly ground black pepper
1 tablespoon apple cider vinegar

Heat the vegetable broth in a large pan and sauté the onion, garlic, and seaweed until tender, about 3 minutes.

Add green and red cabbage, apple, maple syrup, salt, pepper, and vinegar, and cook, covered, over low heat for approximately 20 minutes.

Garnish with fresh fruit.

Yield: 2 servings

EGGPLANT CAPONATA
½ cup vegetable broth
1 large yellow onion, diced
2 cloves garlic, minced
2 stalks celery, sliced
4 tomatoes, chopped
½ cup fresh basil, chopped
2 small eggplants, diced
4 tablespoons pine nuts
2 tablespoons capers, drained
2 tablespoons apple cider vinegar
Sea salt to taste
½ teaspoon freshly ground black pepper

Heat the vegetable broth in a skillet and sauté the onion, garlic, and celery until the onion is translucent.

Add the tomatoes and basil and simmer, covered, for 10 minutes, stirring frequently.

Add the eggplant, pine nuts, capers, vinegar, salt, and pepper, and simmer for 15 minutes.

Serve with toasted bread.

Yields: 4 servings

CREAMY TOFU DIP

2 cups silken tofu
2 tablespoons chopped fresh parsley
2 tablespoons prepared mustard
2 tablespoons apple cider vinegar
2 tablespoons chopped fresh dill (reserve some for garnish)
Sea salt to taste
½ teaspoon freshly ground black pepper
¼ cup chives, chopped

Place the tofu, parsley, mustard, vinegar, dill, salt, pepper, and chives in a food processor or blender and purée until smooth.
Place in a serving dish and garnish with dill.
Serve chilled, with raw vegetables.

Yield: 6 servings

DATE SPREAD

1 cup cooked red kidney beans
2 tablespoons dates, chopped
1 tablespoon fresh mint, chopped
½ cup cashews, chopped
1 tablespoon chia seeds
2 tablespoons grade B maple syrup
1 teaspoon almond extract
1 teaspoon vanilla extract
Sea salt to taste

Purée the beans, dates, and mint in a food processor until smooth.

Add the cashews, chia seeds, maple syrup, almond extract, vanilla extract, and salt, and pulse until well mixed.

Serve with crackers or raw vegetables.

Yield: 5 servings

HOLIDAY STUFFED MUSHROOMS

6 large mushrooms, de-stemmed (mince stems and set aside)
2 tablespoons extra virgin olive oil
1 medium yellow onion, diced
2 cloves garlic, minced
1 red bell pepper, chopped
2 tablespoons flaxseed, ground
2 teaspoons fresh parsley, chopped
½ teaspoon fresh sage, chopped
½ teaspoon fresh rosemary, chopped
½ teaspoon fresh thyme
Sea salt to taste
½ teaspoon freshly ground black pepper
1 tablespoon fresh chives, chopped, for garnish

Preheat oven to 350°F.

Place the mushroom caps on a baking sheet sprayed with nonstick olive oil and bake for 15 minutes, or until brown.

Heat olive oil in a skillet and sauté onion, garlic, and red pepper until the onion is translucent.

Place the minced mushroom stems, onion, garlic, red pepper, flaxseed, parsley, sage, rosemary, thyme, salt, and pepper in a food processor and pulse until coarsely chopped.

Stuff mushroom caps with filling and garnish with chives.

Yield: 6 servings

SPICY TOMATO SALSA

1 cup fresh tomatoes, chopped
¼ cup red onion, chopped
1 tablespoon fresh parsley, chopped
4 tablespoons fresh basil, chopped
1 teaspoon ginger, chopped
1 teaspoon extra virgin olive oil
2 tablespoons fresh hot peppers, minced
Sea salt to taste
½ teaspoon freshly ground black pepper

Combine all the ingredients in a medium bowl and mix until well blended.

Serve with vegetable chips or raw vegetables.

Yield: 6 servings

SPICY BULGUR SALAD

Dressing:
2 tablespoons walnut oil
1 tablespoon raw, unfiltered apple cider vinegar
1 clove garlic, pressed
Sea salt to taste
½ teaspoon freshly ground black pepper
Pinch of cayenne

Salad:
1 cup bulgur, cooked
1 cup spinach, coarsely chopped
1 jar marinated artichoke hearts, quartered
1 tablespoon fresh basil, chopped

½ teaspoon curry powder

½ cup alfalfa sprouts, for garnish

Whisk oil, vinegar, garlic, salt, pepper, and cayenne together in a small bowl.

Place bulgur, spinach, artichoke hearts, basil, and curry powder in a salad bowl and toss the salad with the dressing. Garnish with alfalfa sprouts.

Yield: 2 servings

Breakfasts

AMARANTH PEACH DELIGHT

2 cups water

1 cup amaranth

1 teaspoon chia seeds

½ cup dried peaches, chopped

¼ cup raisins

½ cup pecans, chopped

½ teaspoon ground cinnamon

¼ teaspoon ground cloves

¼ teaspoon ground nutmeg

2 teaspoons pecans, chopped, for garnish

Combine water, amaranth, and chia seeds in a medium saucepan and bring to a slow boil over medium heat.

After 15 minutes, add the dried peaches, raisins, pecans, cinnamon, cloves, and nutmeg, and cook to desired consistency. Garnish with pecans.

Yield: 2 servings

BLUEBERRY-APRICOT OATMEAL

1 cup water
¾ cup steel-cut oats
1 tablespoon chia seeds
1 teaspoon ground cinnamon
½ teaspoon ground ginger
½ cup fresh blueberries
½ cup sliced apricot
½ banana, sliced
¼ cup berries, for garnish

Bring water to a boil in a medium saucepan, add the steel-cut oats, chia seeds, cinnamon, ginger, blueberries, and apricot slices, and reduce heat.

Simmer 5–8 minutes to desired consistency, stirring frequently. Garnish with sliced banana and berries.

Yield: 2 servings

HAWAIIAN RICE CEREAL

¼ cup shredded unsweetened coconut, for garnish
½ cup chopped macadamia nuts
½ cup apple or other fresh juice
1 banana, sliced
½ cup pitted fresh cherries, chopped
½ cup fresh pineapple, chopped
2 cups cooked brown rice
1 teaspoon flax seeds, raw or toasted

Preheat oven to 375°F.

Place unsweetened coconut and macadamia nuts on an ungreased baking pan and bake for 3–5 minutes or until light brown.

In a medium saucepan combine the apple juice, banana, cherries, and pineapple and cook over low heat for 3–5 minutes.

Stir in the brown rice, flax seeds, and macadamia nuts and cook for an additional 2 minutes.

Garnish with toasted coconut.

Yield: 2 servings

BANANA COCONUT BUCKWHEAT CEREAL

½ cup uncooked cream of buckwheat cereal
¼ cup flaxseed meal
2½ cups water
1 tablespoon dried apricots
1 tablespoon dried currants
1 tablespoon raisins
1½ teaspoons ground cinnamon
½ cup banana, sliced
¼ cup toasted coconut flakes

Combine cream of buckwheat, flaxseed meal, and water in a medium saucepan and bring to a slow boil over medium heat.

Add the apricots, currants, raisins, and cinnamon, and cook 5–8 minutes to desired consistency, stirring frequently.

Garnish with sliced banana and coconut.

Yield: 2 servings

COCONUT NUT RICE

1 cup brown rice, cooked
½ cup toasted coconut flakes (save half for garnish)
½ cup cashews, chopped
½ cup dried apricots, chopped, for garnish
1 teaspoon chia seeds
1 teaspoon ground cinnamon
½ teaspoon ground nutmeg
¼ cup all-natural apple juice
¼ cup sunflower seeds, for garnish

Combine brown rice with coconut, cashews, apricots, chia seeds, cinnamon, and nutmeg in a medium bowl.
Place half the mixture and the apple juice in a food processor and pulse until coarsely ground.
Add back to the rest of the rice and mix well.
Garnish with sunflower seeds, apricot pieces and coconut.

Yield: 2 servings

Soups

MISO TOFU SOUP

1 tablespoon walnut oil
4 scallions, sliced
2 cloves garlic, minced
1 large celery stalk, sliced
4 cups water
1 package firm tofu, diced
½ red bell pepper, chopped
½ yellow bell pepper, chopped

3 tablespoons fresh parsley, chopped (save half for garnish)
½ teaspoon oregano
Sea salt to taste
½ teaspoon freshly ground black pepper
4 tablespoons brown rice miso

Heat the oil in a large saucepan and sauté the scallions, garlic, and celery until tender, about 2 minutes.
Add the water, tofu, red and yellow bell pepper, parsley, oregano, salt, and pepper, and simmer for 10 minutes.
Remove 1 cup of hot liquid, dissolve the miso in it, return it to the saucepan, and blend well.
Garnish with parsley.

Yield: 2 servings

PORTUGUESE KALE POTATO SOUP
1 tablespoon olive oil
1 yellow onion, diced
3 cloves garlic, minced
4 cups water
2 cups fresh kale, chopped (reserve 1 tablespoon for garnish)
1 large Yukon gold potato, peeled and cut into cubes
Sea salt to taste
Freshly ground black pepper to taste
Pinch of nutmeg
3 teaspoons spearmint leaves, chopped
1 teaspoon paprika, for garnish

Heat the oil in a large saucepan and sauté the onion and garlic until the onion is translucent.

Add the water, kale, potato, salt, pepper, nutmeg, and spearmint, and cook over medium heat for 15 minutes.

Remove the potato from the soup, place the potato in a blender or food processor with some of the cooking liquid, and purée until smooth.

Return the puréed potato to the soup and stir until well blended.

Garnish with chopped kale and paprika.

Yield: 2 servings

TURNIP AND BLACK BEAN SOUP

1 tablespoon olive oil
1 yellow onion, diced
2 cloves garlic, minced
2 cups black beans, cooked
4 cups water
1 large turnip, diced
Kernels from 1 ear of fresh corn
1 teaspoon fresh thyme, chopped
½ teaspoon cumin
1 bay leaf
Sea salt to taste
½ teaspoon freshly ground black pepper
¼ teaspoon cayenne
2 tablespoons chives, minced, for garnish

Heat the oil in a large saucepan and sauté the onion and garlic until the onion is translucent.

Add the black beans, water, turnip, corn, thyme, cumin, bay leaf, salt, pepper, and cayenne and simmer over low heat for 20 minutes.

Garnish with chives.

Yield: 4 servings

ALGERIAN CHILI
1 tablespoon olive oil
1 medium yellow onion, diced
4 cloves garlic, minced
2 scallions, chopped (reserve 1 tablespoon for garnish)
1 stalk celery, chopped
4 cups water or vegetable broth
1 tomato, coarsely chopped
1 small dried red chili pepper
1 red bell pepper, chopped
½ tablespoon sweet paprika
1 tablespoon curry powder
½ cup tomato paste
2 teaspoons ground cumin
3 cups navy beans, cooked
1 bay leaf
Pinch of cayenne
3 tablespoons fresh parsley, chopped (reserve 1 tablespoon
    for garnish)
Sea salt to taste
½ teaspoon freshly ground black pepper

Heat the oil in a large saucepan and sauté the onion, garlic, scallions, and celery until the onion is translucent.

Add the water, tomato, chili pepper, red bell pepper, paprika, curry powder, tomato paste, and cumin, and simmer until the mixture thickens, stirring frequently.

Add the beans, bay leaf, cayenne, parsley, salt, and pepper, and simmer for 15 minutes.

Garnish with parsley and scallions.

Yield: 4 servings

ITALIAN-STYLE PINTO BEAN SOUP

2 tablespoons olive oil
1 yellow onion, diced
2 cloves garlic, minced
1 stalk celery, chopped
1 red bell pepper, chopped
4 cups water
2 cups pinto beans, cooked
2 carrots, sliced
1 cup mushrooms, sliced
½ cup arugula, chopped
½ teaspoon cumin
Sea salt to taste
½ teaspoon freshly ground black pepper

Heat the oil in a large saucepan and sauté the onion, garlic, celery, and red pepper until the onion is translucent.

Add water, beans, carrots, mushrooms, arugula, cumin, salt, and pepper, and simmer over medium heat for 20 minutes.

Yield: 4 servings

FAVORITE VEGETABLE SOUP

2 tablespoons walnut oil
1 yellow onion, diced
2 cloves garlic, diced
1 stalk celery, sliced (reserve a few slices for garnish)
4 cups vegetable broth
1 cup mung beans, cooked
½ red cabbage, sliced
1 tablespoon chopped fresh parsley
½ teaspoon ground oregano
2 tablespoons fresh basil, chopped
1 tablespoon fresh thyme, chopped
Sea salt to taste
½ teaspoon freshly ground black pepper
1 sprig thyme for garnish
1 cup basmati or brown rice, cooked

Heat the oil in a large saucepan and sauté the onion, garlic, and celery until the onion is translucent.

Add vegetable broth, mung beans, cabbage, parsley, oregano, basil, thyme, salt, and pepper, and cook over medium heat for 15 minutes.

Place soup contents in a blender or food processor and purée. Return the purée to the saucepan, stir in the rice, and cook until thoroughly heated.

Garnish with celery and thyme.

Yield: 4 servings

Entrees

APPLE, WALNUT, AND TOFU SALAD
Dressing:
2 tablespoons walnut oil
1 tablespoon lemon juice
1 clove garlic, minced
Sea salt to taste
½ teaspoon freshly ground black pepper
Pinch cayenne

Salad:
½ cup red onion, diced
1 stalk celery, sliced
¼ teaspoon ground cumin
1 Granny Smith apple, diced
1 package firm tofu, diced
½ cup walnuts
½ cup chives

Whisk oil, lemon juice, garlic, salt, pepper, and cayenne together in a small bowl.
Place onion, celery, cumin, apple, tofu, and walnuts in a salad bowl and toss with the dressing.
Garnish with chives.

Yield: 2 servings

BROCCOLI CAULIFLOWER WITH SHIITAKE MUSHROOMS
¾ cup unsweetened almond milk

1 tablespoon oat flour

1 tablespoon flaxseed meal

1 tablespoon grated lemon zest

1 clove garlic, minced

1 scallion, chopped

1 tablespoon fresh oregano, chopped

1 tablespoon fresh thyme, chopped

1 tablespoon fresh basil, chopped

Sea salt to taste

½ teaspoon freshly ground black pepper

¼ teaspoon cayenne

1 head broccoli, separated into florets

½ head cauliflower, separated into florets

½ cup shiitake mushrooms, chopped

1 cup extra-firm tofu, diced

½ red bell pepper, chopped

½ cup grated vegan cheese

Preheat oven to 325°F.

Whisk together almond milk, flour, flaxseed meal, lemon zest, garlic, scallion, oregano, thyme, basil, salt, pepper, and cayenne in a small bowl.

Combine the broccoli, cauliflower, mushrooms, tofu, and red pepper in a mixing bowl.

Lightly grease a baking dish with olive oil, and add the broccoli mixture.

Pour the almond milk sauce evenly over the vegetables.

Sprinkle with vegan cheese and bake until the sauce thickens, approximately 25 minutes.

Yields: 2–4 servings

BROWN RICE WITH PEPPERS AND HERBS

1 tablespoon walnut oil
1 medium yellow onion, chopped
2 cloves garlic, minced
½ red bell pepper, diced
½ yellow bell pepper, diced
½ green bell pepper, diced
1½ cups brown rice, cooked
¾ tablespoon fresh parsley, chopped
½ teaspoon fresh tarragon, chopped
Sea salt to taste
Freshly ground black pepper to taste
¼ cup arugula
½ cup cherry tomatoes

Heat the oil in a large saucepan and sauté the onion and garlic until the onion is translucent.
Add the peppers and sauté for a minute or two.
Add the rice, parsley, tarragon, salt, and pepper and sauté for 3–5 minutes.
Garnish with arugula and sliced cherry tomatoes.

Yield: 2 servings

CAULIFLOWER WITH GARLIC HUMMUS SAUCE

1 cup chickpeas, cooked
3 tablespoons tahini
2 cloves garlic, minced
1 teaspoon lemon juice
Sea salt to taste
½ teaspoon freshly ground pepper

¼ teaspoon cayenne

1 cup cauliflower florets

1 cup red bell pepper, chopped

1 small red onion, diced

3 tablespoons fresh parsley, chopped (reserve 1 tablespoon for garnish)

¼ teaspoon turmeric

½ cup unsalted whole cashews

2 cups rice, cooked

Preheat oven to 425°F.

Place chickpeas, tahini, garlic, lemon juice, salt, pepper, and cayenne in a food processor and purée until smooth.

In a mixing bowl, combine the chickpea purée, cauliflower, red bell pepper, red onion, parsley, turmeric, and cashews and mix well.

Pour the mixture into a lightly greased, 9-inch by 12-inch baking dish and cover with foil.

Bake for 15–20 minutes, or until the cauliflower is tender.

Serve over rice.

Garnish with parsley.

Yield: 2 servings

BRUSSELS SPROUTS CREOLE

2 tablespoons olive oil

1 large yellow onion, diced

2 garlic cloves, minced

½ red bell pepper, chopped

½ orange bell pepper, chopped

1 fresh tomato, chopped

½ cup water
2 tablespoons fresh basil, chopped
2 tablespoons fresh parsley, chopped
¼ cup olives, pitted and sliced
1 tablespoon grated lemon zest
Sea salt to taste
½ teaspoon freshly ground black pepper
2 cups brussels sprouts, steamed
½ head red leaf lettuce

Heat the oil in a medium saucepan and sauté the onion, garlic, and bell peppers until the onion is translucent.

Add the tomato, water, basil, parsley, olives, lemon zest, salt, and pepper and let simmer for 15 minutes, stirring occasionally.

Add the brussels sprouts and simmer for a few minutes until warm.

Serve on a bed of red leaf lettuce.

Yield: 4–6 servings

BUTTERNUT SQUASH WITH TOASTED SESAME SAUCE

1 butternut squash, peeled and cut into ½-inch pieces
1 tablespoon toasted sesame oil
3 tablespoons tahini
1 clove garlic, minced
2 tablespoons fresh parsley, chopped, divided
Sea salt to taste
½ teaspoon freshly ground pepper
2 tablespoons gomasio
¼ cup sesame seeds
½ cup baby mesclun

Steam the squash for 15–20 minutes until tender.
Remove from the heat and place in individual dishes.
Whisk together the oil, tahini, garlic, half of the parsley, salt, and pepper in a small bowl.
Pour the tahini mixture over the steamed squash.
Sprinkle with gomasio, remaining parsley, and sesame seeds.
Garnish with baby mesclun.

Yield: 2–3 servings

CHICKPEA AND ZUCCHINI CURRY

2 tablespoons olive oil
1 large yellow onion, sliced
4 cloves garlic, minced
1 teaspoon mustard seeds
1 large tomato, chopped
1 can tomato paste
½ cup water
1 tablespoon tamari
2 thin slices of fresh ginger, minced
2 teaspoons turmeric
¼ teaspoon cayenne pepper
2 teaspoons ground cumin
2 teaspoons ground coriander
1 teaspoon ground cinnamon
½ teaspoon ground cloves
Sea salt to taste
½ teaspoon freshly ground black pepper
1 cup chickpeas, cooked
2 medium zucchini, sliced
4–5 cups cooked brown rice
2 tablespoons fresh chives, chopped

Heat the oil in a large skillet and sauté the onion and garlic until the onion is translucent.

Add the mustard seeds and cook until they pop, stirring frequently.

Add the tomato, tomato paste, water, tamari, ginger, turmeric, cayenne, cumin, coriander, cinnamon, cloves, salt, pepper, and chickpeas and stir well.

Cover and simmer for about 15 minutes, stirring frequently.

Add the zucchini, mix well, and let simmer for another 10 minutes.

Serve with brown rice.

Garnish with chives.

Yield: 4–6 servings

CRUNCHY HERBED GREEN BEANS

2 tablespoons olive oil

1 small yellow onion, diced

2 cloves garlic, minced

½ cup green bell pepper

½ cup red bell pepper

½ cup yellow bell pepper

¼ cup water

1 pound green beans, trimmed

½ teaspoon marjoram

1 tablespoon fresh rosemary, chopped

Sea salt to taste

½ teaspoon freshly ground black pepper

Heat the oil in a skillet and sauté the onion, garlic, and peppers until the onions are translucent.

Add the water, green beans, marjoram, rosemary, salt, and pepper and sauté for 3–4 minutes, until the green beans are just tender.

Yield: 4 servings

VEGAN GOULASH
1 tablespoon olive oil
1 medium yellow onion, chopped
2 shallots, minced
2 cloves garlic, minced
1 stalk celery, chopped
1 large tomato, chopped
1 cup vegetable broth
1 package firm tofu, diced
1 cup asparagus, sliced
½ cup chickpeas, cooked
¼ teaspoon caraway seeds
½ teaspoon Hungarian paprika
Sea salt to taste
½ teaspoon freshly ground black pepper
1 tablespoon Bragg's Liquid Aminos
¼ cup tahini

Heat the oil in a large saucepan and sauté the onion, shallots, garlic, and celery until the onion is translucent.
Add tomato and vegetable broth and simmer for 15 minutes.
Add tofu, asparagus, chickpeas, caraway seeds, paprika, salt, and pepper, and simmer for 10 minutes.
Add the Bragg's Liquid Aminos and stir well.
Drizzle with tahini.

Yield: 4 servings

GREEN PEA MILLET COUSCOUS

2 tablespoons walnut oil
2 shallots, minced
2 cloves garlic, minced
1½ cups vegetable broth
¾ cup millet
1 tablespoon chia seeds
½ cup fresh peas
⅓ cup fresh spearmint, chopped
1 tablespoon Bragg's Liquid Aminos, or to taste
½ cup parsley leaves, for garnish
½ teaspoon paprika, for garnish

Heat the oil in a large saucepan and sauté the shallots and garlic for 3 minutes, until tender.

Add the vegetable broth, millet, chia seeds, peas, and spearmint and simmer over low heat for about 15–20 minutes, or until water is absorbed and millet is tender.

Remove from heat and stir in Bragg's Liquid Aminos.

Garnish with parsley and paprika.

Yield: 2 servings

PURPLE CABBAGE AND SPAGHETTI SQUASH STIR-FRY

1 tablespoon olive oil
2 scallions, sliced
3 cloves garlic, minced
2 cups vegetable broth
½ spaghetti squash, diced
2 cups broccoli florets
2 cups purple cabbage, sliced

1 package firm tofu, cubed

1 teaspoon fresh ginger, minced

2 tablespoons fresh parsley, chopped

1 tablespoon fresh thyme, chopped

2 tablespoons tamari

½ teaspoon freshly ground black pepper

¼ cup sesame seeds, for garnish

Heat the oil in a large saucepan and sauté the scallions and garlic until tender.

Add the vegetable broth, squash, broccoli, cabbage, tofu, ginger, parsley, thyme, tamari, and pepper, and simmer for 15–20 minutes until vegetables are tender.

Garnish with the sesame seeds.

Yield: 3 servings

Desserts

BANANA CARAMEL CUSTARD

1 cup almond milk

2 tablespoons arrowroot

2 teaspoons vanilla extract

½ teaspoon almond extract

2 teaspoons ground cinnamon

1 teaspoon ground ginger

½ teaspoon ground nutmeg

1 cup banana, sliced

1 cup maple sugar

1 tablespoon water

In a medium bowl, combine the milk, arrowroot, vanilla extract, almond extract, cinnamon, ginger, and nutmeg and mix well.

Place the mixture in a saucepan over medium heat and simmer, stirring constantly with a whisk or wooden spoon, until thickened.

Once thickened, remove from heat and stir in banana slices.

In a small pan over low flame, combine the maple sugar and water and cook until golden brown.

Pour the sugar mixture evenly into a large, greased ramekin (or 4 individual ramekins).

Add the banana mixture and refrigerate for 2–4 hours.

To serve, gently loosen the pudding from the sides of the dish by running a small knife around the inside of the ramekin.

Place a plate on top of the dish and invert.

(Note: It may be necessary to warm the bottom of the ramekin before inverting, to loosen the pudding.)

Garnish with sliced bananas and a sprinkle of maple sugar and cinnamon.

Yield: 2–4 servings

GOLDEN STRAWBERRY BLUEBERRY CRUMBLE
½ cup spelt flour
½ cup rice flour
1 tablespoon arrowroot
1 cup date sugar, divided
2 tablespoons walnut oil
1 cup fresh or frozen blueberries
1 cup fresh or frozen strawberries
2 teaspoons freshly squeezed lemon juice

1 teaspoon ground cinnamon

1 tablespoon flaked coconut, fresh or packaged

Preheat the oven to 300°F.

In a large bowl, combine the flours, arrowroot, ½ cup date sugar, and walnut oil and blend using a fork or pastry blender.

Place blueberries and strawberries in a soufflé dish and mix in lemon juice, ½ cup date sugar, and cinnamon until berries are well coated.

Cover berries evenly with the crumble mixture.

Place in the oven and bake for 15–20 minutes, or until golden brown.

Yield: 4 servings

CHILLED CANTALOUPE STUFFED WITH CHERRY CREAM

1 cantaloupe

1 cup fresh or frozen cherries, pitted

½ teaspoon lemon extract

½ teaspoon almond extract

2 cups silken tofu

Cut the cantaloupe into quarters and discard seeds. Remove the fruit from the peel and slice into bite-sized pieces.

Combine the cherries, lemon extract, almond extract, and tofu in a food processor or blender and puree until smooth.

Place the cherry cream in a dessert dish and serve with the sliced cantaloupe.

Garnish with sliced lemon.

Yield: 4 servings

Additional Resources

Suggested Reading

- *A Cancer Battle Plan: Six Strategies for Beating Cancer, from a Recovered "Hopeless Case,"* by Anne E. Frahm
- *A Cancer Therapy: Results of Fifty Cases and the Cure of Advanced Cancer,* by Charlotte Gerson
- *A Cancer Therapy: Results of Fifty Cases and the Cure of Advanced Cancer by Diet Therapy: A Summary of 30 Years of Clinical Experimentation,* by Max Gerson
- *A Consumer's Dictionary of Cosmetic Ingredients,* by Ruth Winter
- *Alive & Well: One Doctor's Experience with Nutrition in the Treatment of Cancer Patients,* by Philip E. Binzel
- *Alternative Medicine: The Definitive Guide* (2nd edition), by Burton Goldberg Group
- *Alternatives in Cancer Therapy: The Complete Guide to Non-traditional Treatments,* by Ross Pelton
- *Apple Cider Vinegar—Miracle Health System,* by Paul C. Bragg and Patricia Bragg
- *Aveline Kushi's Complete Guide to Macrobiotic Cooking,* by Aveline Kushi
- *Be a Healthy Woman,* by Gary Null and Amy McDonald

- *Beating Cancer with Nutrition* (revised), by Patrick Quillin and Noreen Quillin
- *Beauty to Die For: The Cosmetic Consequence,* by Judi Vance
- *Cancer and Vitamin C: A Discussion of the Nature, Causes, Prevention, and Treatment of Cancer with Special Reference to the Value of Vitamin C,* by Ewan Cameron and Linus Pauling (contributor)
- *Cancer: Curing the Incurable without Surgery, Chemotherapy, or Radiation,* by William Donald Kelley
- *Cancer Diagnosis: What to Do Next,* by W. John Diamond
- *Cancer-Free: 30 Who Triumphed over Cancer Naturally,* by East West Foundation with Ann Fawcett and Cynthia Smith
- *Cancer Therapy: The Independent Consumer's Guide to Non-toxic Treatment and Prevention,* by Ralph W. Moss
- *Cancer—The Problem and the Solution,* by Dr. Johanna Budwig
- *Cancer—Why We're Still Dying to Know the Truth,* by Phillip Day
- *Censured for Curing Cancer: The American Experience of Dr. Max Gerson,* by Max Gerson
- *Coping with Cancer: How to Prevent and Treat Cancer with Vitamins, Minerals, and Diet,* by Morton Walker
- *Dr. Max Gerson: Healing the Hopeless,* by Max Gerson
- *Drop-Dead Gorgeous: Protecting Yourself from the Hidden Dangers of Cosmetics,* by Kim Erickson
- *Dying to Look Good: The Disturbing Truth about What's Really in Your Cosmetics, Toiletries and Personal Care Products,* by Christine Hoza Farlow

- *Fats and Oils: The Complete Guide to Fats and Oils in Health and Nutrition,* by Udo Erasmus
- *Fighting Cancer with Vitamins and Antioxidants,* by Kedar N. Prasad, PhD, and K. Che Prasad, MS, MD
- *Flax Oil as a True Aid against Arthritis, Heart Infarction, Cancer, and Other Diseases,* by Dr. Johanna Budwig
- *Flood Your Body with Oxygen,* by Ed McCabe
- *Gerson Diet Therapy for Women's Cancers: Breast Cancer, Ovarian Cancer, Cervical Cancer,* by Charlotte Gerson
- *Get Healthy Now,* by Gary Null
- *Healing Cancer,* by Michio Kushi
- *Healing outside the Margins: The Survivor's Guide to Integrative Cancer Care,* by Carole O'Toole and Carolyn B. Hendricks, MD
- *Health and Nutrition Secrets That Can Save Your Life,* by Russell L. Blaylock, MD
- *Health Wars,* by Phillip Day
- *Heinerman's Encyclopedia of Healing Juices,* by John Heinerman
- *How I Conquered Cancer Naturally,* by Eydie Mae and Chris Loeffler
- *How to Fight Cancer & Win,* by William L. Fischer
- *How to Prevent Breast Cancer,* by Ross Pelton
- *Hydrogen Peroxide: Medical Miracle,* by William Campbell Douglass
- *Hyperbaric Oxygen Therapy,* by Morton Walker
- *Introduction to Oxygen Therapies: Is This the Answer to Colds, Flu, AIDS, Cancer and Most Other Diseases?,* by Ed McCabe
- *Living Well Naturally,* by Anthony J. Sattilaro

- *Mind, Body, and Soul: A Guide to Living with Cancer,* by Nancy Hassett Dahm
- *My Beautiful Life: How Macrobiotics Brought Me from Cancer to Radiant Health,* by Milenka Dobic
- *Natural Hygiene: Man's Pristine Way of Life,* by Dr. Herbert M. Shelton
- *O2Xygen O2xygen Therapies: A New Way of Approaching Disease,* by Ed McCabe
- *One Answer to Cancer,* by William Donald Kelley
- *Options: The Alternative Cancer Therapy Book,* by Richard Walters
- *Oxygen Healing Therapies: For Optimum Health & Vitality: Bio-Oxidative Therapies for Treating Immune Disorders, Candida, Cancer, Heart, Skin, Circulatory, and Other Modern Diseases,* by Nathaniel Altman
- *Questioning Chemotherapy: A Critique of the Use of Toxic Drugs in the Treatment of Cancer,* by Ralph W. Moss
- *Recalled by Life,* by Anthony J. Sattilaro
- *Return to Wholeness: Embracing Body, Mind, and Spirit in the Face of Cancer,* by Deepak Chopra
- *Safer Medicine,* by Mayer Eisenstein
- *The Breuss Cancer Cure: Advice for the Prevention and Natural Treatment of Cancer, Leukemia and Other Seemingly Incurable Diseases,* by Rudolf Breuss
- *The Burzynski Breakthrough,* by Thomas D. Elias
- *The Cancer Cure That Worked: 50 Years of Suppression,* by Barry Lynes
- *The Cancer Industry: The Classic Exposé on the Cancer Establishment,* by Ralph W. Moss

- *The Cancer Prevention Diet: Michio Kushi's Macrobiotic Blueprint for the Prevention and Relief of Disease,* by Michio Kushi with Alex Jack
- *The Cancer Survival Cookbook: 200 Quick & Easy Recipes with Helpful Eating Hints,* by Donna L. Weihofen
- *The Complete Book of Enzyme Therapy,* by Anthony Cichoke
- *The Complete Encyclopedia of Natural Healing,* by Gary Null
- *The Cure for All Advanced Cancers,* by Hulda Regehr Clark
- *The Cure for All Cancers,* by Dr. Hulda Clark
- *The Cure for All Cancers: Including over 100 Case Histories of Persons Cured,* by Hulda Clark
- *The Gerson Therapy: The Amazing Nutritional Program for Cancer and Other Illnesses,* by Charlotte Gerson
- *The Hippocrates Diet and Health Program,* by Ann Wigmore
- *The Juicing Bible,* by Pat Crocker and Susan Eagles
- *The Macrobiotic Approach to Cancer: Towards Preventing and Controlling Cancer with Diet and Lifestyle,* by Michio Kushi
- *The Miracle of Fasting: Proven throughout History for Physical, Mental and Spiritual Rejuvenation,* by Paul C. Bragg and Patricia Bragg
- *The Miraculous Diet: A New Era in Health & Well-Being: The Revolutionary Discoveries of Max Gerson, M.D.,* by Max Gerson
- *The Prostate: A Guide for Men and the Women Who Love Them,* Patrick C. Walsh, MD, and Janet Farrar Worthington

- *The Safe Shopper's Bible: A Consumer's Guide to Nontoxic Household Products,* by David Steinman and Samuel S. Epstein
- *The Shocking Truth about Water,* by Paul C. Bragg and Patricia Bragg
- *The What to Eat If You Have Cancer Cookbook,* by Daniella Chace and Maureen Keane
- *Tomato Power: Lycopene: The Miracle Nutrient That Can Prevent Aging, Heart Disease and Cancer,* by James F. Balch
- *Ultimate Juicing: Delicious Recipes for over 125 of the Best Fruit and Vegetable Juice Combinations,* by Donna Pliner Rodnitzky
- *What to Eat If You Have Cancer,* by Daniella Chace and Maureen Keane
- *When Hope Never Dies: One Woman's Remarkable Recovery from Cancer—and the Natural Program That Saved Her Life,* by Tom Monte
- *World without Cancer: The Story of Vitamin B17,* by G. Edward Griffin
- *Your Face Never Lies: Introduction to Oriental Diagnosis,* by Michio Kushi

Suggested Documentaries

- *Burzynski: The Movie,* by Eric Mercola
- *Cut, Poison, Burn,* by Wayne Chesler
- *Dying to Have Known,* by Steve Kroschel
- *Healing Cancer,* by Mike Anderson
- *Pink Ribbons, Inc.,* by Lea Pool
- *Preventing and Reversing Cancer Naturally,* by Gary Null

- *The Beautiful Truth,* by Steve Kroschel
- *The Gerson Miracle,* by Steve Kroschel

About the Author

Dr. Gary Null is the host of the nation's longest-running public radio program on nutrition and alternative medicine and an award-winning director of progressive documentary films, including *Autism: Made in the USA* (2009) and *Death by Medicine* (2011).

Managing Editor—Jeremy Stillman
Editor—Max W. Kortlander

Endnotes

[1] American Cancer Society. Cancer Facts & Figures 2016. Atlanta: American Cancer Society, 2016.

[2] "41 Percent of Americans Will Get Cancer." UPI.com. Accessed March 2, 2012. http://www.upi.com/Health_News/2010/05/06/41-percent-of-Americans-will-get-cancer/UPI-75711273192042/.

[3] American Cancer Society. Cancer Facts & Figures 2016.

[4] Epstein, Samuel S. *National Cancer Institute and American Cancer Society: Criminal Indifference to Cancer Prevention and Conflicts of Interest*. Self-published manuscript. United States: Xlibris Corporation, 2011.

[5] Ibid.

[6] Ibid.

[7] Pierce, Tanya Harter. *Outsmart Your Cancer: Alternative Non-toxic Treatments That Work*. 2nd ed. Stateline, NV: Thoughtworks Publishing, 2009.

[8] "How the Losing Cancer War Is Being Spun Warns Samuel S. Epstein, M.D." PR Newswire. Accessed January 16, 2012. http://www.prnewswire.com/news-releases/how-the-losing-cancer-war-is-being-spun-warns-samuel-s-epstein-md-and-quentin-d-young-md-71761482.html.

[9] "FY 2016 Budget." National Cancer Institute. http://www.cancer.gov/about-nci/budget/congressional-justification/fy2016-nci-congressional-justification.pdf.

[10] Epstein, *Criminal Indifference to Cancer Prevention*.

[11] "FY 2016 Budget." National Cancer Institute.

[12] "Letter to Senate Committee on Health, Education, Labor and Pensions." preventcancer.com. Accessed January 23, 2012.

[13] Ibid.

[14] Ho, Dr. Mae-Wan. "Cancer: An Epigenetic Disease." The Institute of Science in Society. Accessed April 5, 2012. http://www.i-sis.org.uk/Cancer_an_Epigenetic_Disease.php.

[15] Rubin, Harry, and Bryan Ellison. "Individual Transforming Events in Long-Term Cell Culture of NIH 3T3 Cells as Products of Epigenetic Induction." *Cancer Research* 52 (1992). Accessed April 2, 2012. http://cancerres.aacrjournals.org/content/52/3/667.full.pdf.

[16] Ho, "Cancer: An Epigenetic Disease."

[17] Ibid.

[18] Epstein, *Criminal Indifference to Cancer Prevention.*

[19] Ibid.

[20] Ibid.

[21] Epstein, "American Cancer Society."

[22] "Recombinant Bovine Growth Hormone." American Cancer Society. Accessed January 31, 2012. http://www.cancer.org/cancer/cancercauses/othercarcinogens/athome /recombinant-bovine-growth-hormone.

[23] Israel, Brett. "How Many Cancers Are Caused by the Environment?" *Scientific American* (May 21, 2010). Accessed February 8, 2012. http://www.scientificamerican .com/article.cfm?id=how-many-cancers-are-caused-by-the-environment.

[24] Davis, Devra Lee. *The Secret History of the War on Cancer.* New York: Basic Books, 2009.

[25] Epstein, Samuel. "Samuel S. Epstein: The American Cancer Society Trivializes Cancer Risks: Blatant Conflicts of Interest." *Huffington Post.* Accessed January 23, 2012. http:// www.huffingtonpost.com/samuel-s-epstein/the-american-cancer-socie_b_568292.html.

[26] "The American Cancer Society: The World's Wealthiest 'Nonprofit' Institution." Cancer Prevention Coalition. Accessed January 23, 2012.

[27] Ibid.

[28] Ibid.

[29] "Charity Navigator Rating—American Cancer Society." Charity Navigator. Accessed January 19, 2012. http://www.charitynavigator.org/index.cfm?bay=search .summary&orgid=6495.

[30] Ibid.

[31] Ibid.

[32] "Charity Navigator Rating."

[33] Epstein, *Criminal Indifference to Cancer Prevention.*

[34] Ibid.

[35] Marchione, Marilynn. "Taxol May Be Ineffective for Many Cancer Patients." redOrbit. Accessed March 19, 2012.

[36] Ibid.

[37] "Still Losing," World-Wire.

[38] Epstein, Samuel S. "President Obama and the Congress Must Take Action on Cancer Prevention." *Huffington Post.* Acessed March 19, 2012. http://www.huffington post. com/samuel-s-epstein/president-obama-and-the-c_b_435547.html.

[39] Tara Parker-Pope. "Mammogram's Role as a Savior Is Tested." *New York Times,* October 24, 2011.

[40] Kruk, J., and Aboul-Enein, H. Y. "Psychological Stress and the Risk of Breast Cancer: A Case-Control Study." *Cancer Detection and Prevention* 28, no. 6 (2004): 399–408.

[41] Prate, Dawn. "Mammograms Cause Breast Cancer (and Other Cancer Facts You Probably Never Knew." Natural News. Accessed October 1, 2013. http://www.naturalnews .com/010886.html.

[42] Kawa, Lucas. "Regular Doctor's Check-Ups Are a Big Waste of Money." Business Insider. Accessed October 1, 2013. http://www.businessinsider.com/check-ups-dont-improve-health-outcomes-2013-1.

[43] Welch, H. G., and B. A. Frankel. "Likelihood That a Woman with Screen-Detected Breast Cancer Has Had Her 'Life Saved' by That Screening." *Archives of Internal Medicine* 171, no. 22 (December 12, 2011).

[44] Wright, C. J., and C. B. Mueller. "Screening Mammography and Public Health Policy: The Need for Perspective." *The Lancet* 346, no. 8966 (July 1, 1995): 29–32.

[45] Welch, H. "The Sea of Uncertainty Surrounding Ductal Carcinoma in Situ—the Price of Screening Mammography." *Journal of the National Cancer Institute* 100, no. 4: 228–29.

[46] "Thermography Is a Safe Alternative to Mammography." Natural Health News. Accessed February 2, 2012. http://www.naturalnews.com/033586_thermography _mammography.html.

[47] Ibid.

[48] Gøtzsche, P. C., and K. J. Jørgensen. "Screening for Breast Cancer with Mammography." *Cochrane Database Syst Rev* (June 4, 2013): CD001877.

[49] Wright and Mueller, "Screening Mammography."

[50] Epstein, Samuel. "Corporate Sponsors Control Mammography Industry Warns Cancer Prevention Coalition." World-Wire. Accessed February 3, 2012.

[51] Gale, Jason. "Prostate Exam Deaths From 'Superbugs' Spur Inquiry into Cancer Tests." Bloomberg. Accessed February 1, 2012. http://www.bloomberg.com/news/2011-05-05/prostate-exam-deaths-tied-to-superbug-ills-spur-cancer-test-inquiries.html.

[52] Ibid.

[53] Gordon, Serena. "Prostate Biopsies Can Raise Risk of Hospitalization." USATODAY. com. Accessed February 1, 2012.

[54] Sandblom et al. "Randomised Prostate Cancer Screening Trial: 20-Year Follow-Up." *British Medical Journal* 342 (2011): d1539. Accessed January 18, 2012. http://www.bmj.com/content/342/bmj.d1539.

[55] Schröder et al. "Screening and Prostate-Cancer Mortality in a Randomized European Study." *The New England Journal of Medicine* 360 (2009): 1320–28. Accessed January 23, 2012. http://www.nejm.org/doi/full/10.1056/NEJMoa0810084.

[56] Ibid.

[57] "Setback Reported in Research into Cancer Treatment." BostonHerald.com. Accessed March 9, 2012.

[58] University of Michigan Comprehensive Cancer Center. "50 is the Golden Age to Begin Routine Colonoscopies." Accessed August 4, 2013.

[59] US Multisociety Task Force on Colorectal Cancer et al. "Colorectal Cancer Screening and Surveillance." Accessed August 20, 2013. https://www.med.upenn.edu/gastro /documents/AGAtechnicalreviewcolorectalcancerscreening.pdf.

[60] Atkin, W. S., and B. P. Saunders. "Surveillance Guidelines after Removal of Colorectal Adenomatous Polyps." Accessed August 20, 2013. http://gut.bmj.com/content/51 /suppl_5/v6.full.pdf.

[61] WebMD. "Colonoscopy." Accessed August 20, 2013. http://www.webmd.com /colorectal-cancer/colonoscopy-16695.

[62] UK Department for Work and Pensions. "Tests for Bowel Cancer Including Rectal Cancer." Accessed August 20, 2013.

[63] Levin, T. R., W. Zhao, C. Conell, L. C. Seeff, D. L. Manninen, J. A. Shapiro, J. Schulman. "Complications of Colonoscopy in an Integrated Health Care Delivery System." *Annals of Internal Medicine* 145, no. 12 (December 19, 2006): 880–86.

[64] Johns Hopkins Medicine. "Colonoscopy." Accessed August 20, 2013. http://www .hopkinsmedicine.org/healthlibrary/test_procedures/gastroenterology/colonoscopy _92,P07693/.

[65] Rabenecket, L., et al. "Bleeding and Perforation after Outpatient Colonoscopy and Their Risk Factors in Usual Clinical Practice." Accessed August 20, 2013. http://www.ncbi .nlm.nih.gov/pubmed/18938166.

[66] Cohen, Lawrence, David M. Kastenberg, David B. Mount, and Alan V. Safdi. "Current Issues in Optimal Bowel Preparation." Accessed August 20, 2013.

[67] Mercola, Joseph. "Can Colon Cancer Screenings Cause More Harm Than Good?" Accessed February 2, 2012. http://articles.mercola.com/sites/articles/archive/2008/01/10 /can-colon-cancer-screenings-cause-more-harm-than-good.aspx.

[68] "Study: Many Elderly Get Colon Screening Too Often." Yahoo! Health. Accessed February 2, 2012.

[69] "Setback Reported," BostonHerald.com.

[70] Ibid.

[71] "Questions about Chemotherapy." American Cancer Society. Accessed March 9, 2012. http://www.cancer.org/Treatment/TreatmentsandSideEffects/TreatmentTypes /Chemotherapy/WhatItIsHowItHelps/chemo-what-it-is-questions-about-chemo.

[72] Moss, Ralph W. *Questioning Chemotherapy.* Brooklyn, NY: Equinox Press, 1995.

[73] Ibid.

[74] "The Contribution of Cytotoxic Chemotherapy to 5-Year Survival in Adult Malignancies." *Clinical Oncology (Royal College of Radiologists (Great Britain))* 16, no. 8 (December 2004): 549–60. Accessed March 5, 2012. http://www.ncbi.nlm.nih .gov/pubmed/15630849.

[75] "Chemotherapy Statistics Can Be Misleading." Scientific Living. Accessed March 6, 2012.

[76] "NCEPOD—SACT: For Better, for Worse? Report (2008)." National Confidential Enquiry into Patient Outcome and Death. Accessed March 5, 2012.

[77] Ibid.

[78] Lavie, O., O. Barnett-Griness, S. A. Narod, G. Rennert. "The Risk of Developing Uterine Sarcoma after Tamoxifen Use." *International Journal of Gynecological Cancer* (2007). Wiley Online Library. Accessed March 6, 2012.

[79] Smith, Carol. "Lifesaving Drugs May Be Killing Health Workers." *Seattle Times.* Accessed February 28, 2012.

[80] "Law Would Level the Playing Field for Chemotherapy Pills." RVANews. Accessed March 5, 2012. http://rvanews.com/news/law-would-level-the-playing-field-for-chemotherapy-pills/57342.

[81] Marchione, Marilynn. "Provenge, Cancer Drug, Costs $93,000: Sky-High Drug Prices Impact Life-or-Death Decisions." *Huffington Post*. Accessed March 6, 2012.

[82] "Law Would Level," RVANews.

[83] Ibid.

[84] Edwards, Jim. "Why a $93,000 Cancer Drug Can't Shake off Rumors It Doesn't Work." CBS News. Accessed March 6, 2012. http://www.cbsnews.com/8301-505123_162-42845241/why-a-93000-cancer-drug-cant-shake-off-rumors-it-doesnt-work/?tag=bnetdomain.

[85] "NCEPOD—SACT," National Confidential Enquiry into Patient Outcome and Death.

[86] Pollack, Andrew. "Heated, Harrowing Chemotherapy Bath May Be Only Hope for Some." *New York Times*. Accessed February 28, 2012. http://www.nytimes.com/2011/08/12/business/heated-chemotherapy-bath-may-be-only-hope-for-some-cancer-patients.html.

[87] Ibid.

[88] Ausubel, Ken. *When Healing Becomes a Crime: The Amazing Story of the Hoxsey Cancer Clinics and the Return of Alternative Therapies*. Rochester, VT: Healing Arts Press, 2000.

[89] "Self-Seeding of Cancer Cells May Play a Critical Role in Tumor Progression." Memorial Sloan Kettering Cancer Center. Accessed March 2, 2012. http://www.mskcc.org/news/press/self-seeding-cells-may-play-critical-role-tumor-progression.

[90] Grady, Denise. "Repeat Breast Cancer Surgery Guidelines Found Unclear." *New York Times*. Accessed February 28, 2012. http://www.nytimes.com/2012/02/01/health/repeat-breast-cancer-surgery-guidelines-found-unclear.html?_r=1&scp=2&sq=breast percent20cancer&st=cse.

[91] Olaya, Windy, John W. Morgan, Sharon S. Lum. "Unnecessary Axillary Surgery for Patients with Node-Negative Breast Cancer Undergoing Total Mastectomy." Abstract. *Archives of Surgery* 146, no. 9 (September 2011): 1029. Accessed March 2, 2012. http://archsurg.ama-assn.org/cgi/content/abstract/146/9/1029.

[92] Grady, Denise. "Lymph Node Study Shakes Pillar of Breast Cancer Care." *New York Times*. Accessed March 2, 2012. http://www.nytimes.com/2011/02/09/health/research/09breast.html?pagewanted=all.

[93] Ibid.

[94] Griffin, G. Edward. *World without Cancer*. Westlake Village, CA: American Media, 2000.

[95] Faloon, William. "Cancer Establishment Hides Radiation Side Effects." Life Extension. Accessed March 7, 2012. http://www.lef.org/magazine/mag2011/dec2011_Cancer-Establishment-Hides-Radiation-Side-Effects_01.htm.

[96] Ibid.

[97] Ibid.

[98] "Radiation of Left Breast during Cancer Treatment Causes Coronary Artery Disease." Natural Health News. Accessed March 7, 2012. http://www.naturalnews.com/019989_conventional_cancer_treatments_radiation_therapy.html.

99 Gutierrez, David. "Radiation Treatment for Cancer Causes Diabetes in Children." Natural Health News. Accessed March 7, 2012. http://www.naturalnews.com/028032 _radiation_therapy_diabetes.html.

100 Ibid.

101 Samadi, David. "New Dangers of Radiation Therapy Exposed." *Ethiopian News and Opinion Journal*. Accessed March 7, 2012.

102 Ibid.

103 Gripp, S., et al. "Palliative Radiotherapy Tailored to Life Expectancy in End-Stage Cancer Patients." *Cancer* 116, no. 13 (July 1, 2010): 3251.

104 Ibid.

105 Ibid.

106 Smith, B. D., et al. "Adoption of Intensity-Modulated Radiation Therapy for Breast Cancer in the United States." *Journal of the National Cancer Institute* 103, no. 10 (May 18, 2011): 798–809.

107 "NCI Cancer Bulletin for May 3, 2011." National Cancer Institute. Accessed March 8, 2012.

108 Nguyen, Paul, et al. "Cost Implications of the Rapid Adoption of Newer Technologies for Treating Prostate Cancer." *Journal of Clinical Oncology* 31, no. 1217 (2011): 1–11.

109 Ibid.

110 Bao, Bin, et al. "Cancer Stem Cells (CSCs) and Mechanisms of Their Regulation: Implications for Cancer Therapy." Current protocols in pharmacology / editorial board, Eds. S. J. Enna et al. 0 14 (2013): Unit–14.25. Accessed December 4, 2016. doi:10.1002/0471141755.ph1425s61.

111 Visvader, Jane E., and Geoffrey J. Lindeman. "Cancer Stem Cells: Current Status and Evolving Complexities." *Cell Stem Cell* 10, no. 6 (June 14, 2012): 717–28 .doi:10.1016/j.stem.2012.05.007.

112 Yanqing, Huang, Tomoaki Hamana, Junchen Liu, Cong Wang, Lei An, Pan You, et al. "Type 2 Fibroblast Growth Factor Receptor Signaling Preserves Stemness and Prevents Differentiation of Prostate Stem Cells from the Basal Compartment." *Journal of Biological Chemistry* 290, no. 29 (2015): 17753.

113 Pingping, Zhu, Yanying Wang, Jiayi Wu, Guanling Huang, Benyu Liu, Buqing Ye, et al. "LncBRM Initiates YAP1 Signalling Activation to Drive Self-Renewal of Liver Cancer Stem Cells." *Nature Communications* 7, no. 13608 (December 1, 2016).

114 "Cancer Stem Cells." GreenMedInfo. http://www.greenmedinfo.com/disease/cancer -stem-cells.

115 Minton, Barbara. "Marijuana Kills Cancer Cells, Admits the U.S. National Cancer Institute." Natural Society. August 26, 2015. Accessed October 5, 2016. http://natural-society.com/marijuana-kills-cancer-cells-admits-the-u-s-national-cancer-institute/.

116 Singh, Y., and C. Bali. "Cannabis Extract Treatment for Terminal Acute Lymphoblastic Leukemia with a Philadelphia Chromosome Mutation." *Case Reports in Oncology*, no. 3 (2013): 585–92.

117 Wang, J., Y. Deng, Y. Tan, K. Li, B. Wen, Q. Zhao. "Cannabinoid WIN55, 212–2 Inhibits Proliferation, Invasion and Migration of Human SMMC-7721 Hepatocellular

Carcinoma Cells." *Chinese Journal of Cellular and Molecular Immunology* 32, no. 5 (2016): 619–24.

[118] Nabissi, M., et al. "Cannabinoids Synergize with Carfilzomib, Reducing Multiple Myeloma Cells Viability and Migration." *Oncotarget*, October 18, 2016: 12721.

[119] Moreno, E., C. Andradas, M. Medrano, M. M. Caffarel, E. Perez-Gomez, S. Blasco-Benito, et al. "Targeting CB2-GPR55 Receptor Heteromers Modulates Cancer Cell Signaling." *Journal of Biological Chemistry* 289, no. 32 (July 18, 2014): 21960–72. doi:10.1074/jbc.m114.561761.

[120] "Complementary Alternative Cancer Therapies—Conventional Cancer Treatment, Chemotherapy—Life Extension Health Concern." Life Extension. Accessed April 1, 2012. http://www.lef.org/protocols/cancer/alternative_cancer_therapies_01.htm.

[121] Cone, Maria. "President's Cancer Panel: Environmentally Caused Cancers Are 'Grossly Underestimated' and 'Needlessly Devastate American Lives.'" Environmental Health News. Accessed February 15, 2012. http://www.environmentalhealthnews.org/ehs/news/presidents-cancer-panel.

[122] Epstein, Samuel. "Milk: America's Health Problem." Cancer Prevention Coalition. Accessed March 12, 2012.

[123] "AICR Statement: Hot Dogs and Cancer Risk." Medical News Today. Accessed March 12, 2012. http://www.medicalnewstoday.com/releases/158507.php.

[124] Mayo Clinic Staff. "Low White Blood Cell Count." Accessed August 30, 2013. http://www.mayoclinic.com/health/low-white-blood-cell-count/MY00162/DSECTION=causes.

[125] "The 'Dirty Dozen' Consumer Products." Cancer Prevention Coalition. Accessed February 15, 2012.

[126] Gao, Xiang, et al. "Prospective Studies of Dairy Product and Calcium Intakes and Prostate Cancer Risk: A Meta-analysis." *Journal of the National Cancer Institute* 97, no. 23 (2005): 1768–77.

[127] Zhu, G., Y. Q. Zhang, and B. Wan. "Role of Dietary Factors in Prostate Cancer Development." *Zhonghua Nan Ke Xue* 11, no. 5 (May 2005): 375–78

[128] Larsson, S. C., N. Orsini, and A. Wolk. "Milk, Milk Products and Lactose Intake and Ovarian Cancer Risk: A Meta-analysis of Epidemiological Studies." *International Journal of Cancer* 118, no. 2 (January 15, 2006): 431–41.

[129] Chan, J. M., M. J. Stampfer, J. Ma, P. H. Gann, J. M. Gaziano, and E. Giovannucci. "Dairy Products, Calcium, and Prostate Cancer Risk in the Physicians' Health Study." *American Journal of Clinical Nutrition* 74 (2001): 549–54.

[130] "FDA: Some Chicken May Have Small Amount of Arsenic." phillyBurbs.com. Accessed March 12, 2012.

[131] Adams, Mike. "FDA Finally Admits Chicken Meat Contains Cancer-Causing Arsenic (but Keep Eating It, Yo!)." Natural Health News. Accessed March 12, 2012. http://www.naturalnews.com/032659_arsenic_chicken.html.

[132] "Questions and Answers Regarding 3-Nitro (Roxarsone)." US Food and Drug Administration. Accessed March 13, 2012. http://www.fda.gov/AnimalVeterinary/Safety Health/ProductSafetyInformation/ucm258313.htm.

[133] Consumer Reports. "How Much Arsenic Is in Your Rice?" (November 18, 2014).

[134] Ibid.

[135] Ibid.

[136] Moore, Nancy. "Cancer-Causing Foods: 3 Culprits and 6 Top Foods." Natural Healing, Natural Health. Accessed March 12, 2012.

[137] "Annual Report to the Nation Shows Continuing Decline in Cancer Mortality." JNCI. Accessed February 15, 2012. http://jnci.oxfordjournals.org/content/103/9/NP.1.

[138] "CSPI Says Food Dyes Pose Rainbow of Risks." Center for Science in the Public Interest. Accessed February 15, 2012. http://www.cspinet.org/new/201006291.html.

[139] Collaborative Group on Hormonal Factors in Breast Cancer. "Alcohol, Tobacco and Breast Cancer—Collaborative Reanalysis of Individual Data from 53 Epidemiological Studies, Including 58,515 Women with Breast Cancer and 95,067 Women without the Disease." British Journal of Cancer 87, no. 11 (2002):1234–45.

[140] Mulcahy, Nick. "Even Light Alcohol Drinking Ups Breast Cancer Risk: No Safe Level?" Accessed March 30, 2012. http://www.medscape.com/viewarticle/761187.

[141] "Reducing Environmental Cancer Risk." nih.gov. Accessed March 8, 2012. https://deainfo.nci.nih.gov/advisory/pcp/annualreports/pcp08-09rpt/PCP_Report_08-09_508.pdf.

[142] Epstein, Samuel. "Samuel S. Epstein: President's Cancer Panel Warns of Toxic Effects of BPA." Huffington Post. Accessed March 9, 2012. http://www.huffingtonpost.com/samuel-s-epstein/presidents-cancer-panel-w_b_566541.html.

[143] "Reducing Environmental Cancer Risk." nih.gov.

[144] Sandler, D. P., and J. A. Ross. "Epidemiology of Acute Leukemia in Children and Adults." Seminars in Oncology 24 (1997): 3–16.

[145] Mandal, Ananya. "Prostate Cancer Linked to Pesticides: Study." The Medical News. Accessed March 2, 2012. http://www.news-medical.net/news/20110831/Prostate-cancer-linked-to-pesticides-Study.aspx?utm_source=twitterfeed&utm_medium=twitter.

[146] Zahm, S. H., and M. H. Ward. "Pesticides and Childhood Cancer." Environmental Health Perspectives 106, no. S-3 (1998). Accessed March 6, 2012.

[147] "Chlordane." US Environmental Protection Agency. Accessed March 5, 2012.

[148] Pogoda, Preston-Martin. "Household Pesticides and Risk of Pediatric Brain Tumors." Environmental Health Perspectives 105 (1997): 1214–20.

[149] Stanford University. "Even Low Exposure to X-rays, Gamma Rays Increases Cancer Risk, Study Finds." ScienceDaily. October 27, 2005. Accessed April 1, 2012. http://www.sciencedaily.com/releases/2005/10/051027090539.htm.

[150] Feychting, M., G. Schulgen, J. H. Olsen, and A. Ahlbom. "Magnetic Fields and Childhood Cancer—A Pooled Analysis of Two Scandinavian Studies." European Journal of Cancer 31A (1995): 2035–9.

[151] Ahlbom, I. C., E. Cardis, A. Green, M. Linet, D. Savitz, and A. Swerdlow. "Review of the Epidemiologic Literature on EMF and Health." Environmental Health Perspectives 109, suppl. 6 (December 2001): 911–33. doi:10.2307/3454653.

[152] Savitz, D. A., H. Wachtel, F. A. Barnes, E. M. John, and J. G. Tvrdik. "Case-Control Study of Childhood Cancer and Exposure to 60-Hz Magnetic Fields." American Journal of Epidemiology 128 (1988): 21–38.

[153] Bethwaite, P., A. Cook, J. Kennedy, and N. Pearce. "Acute Leukemia in Electrical Workers: A New Zealand Case-Control Study." *Cancer Causes and Control* 12, no. 8 (October 2001): 683–89.

[154] Draper et. al. "Childhood Cancer in Relation to Distance from High Voltage Power Lines in England and Wales: A Case Control Study." *British Medical Journal* 330, no. 7503 (June 4, 2005): 1290.

[155] Bracy, Kate. "Toxic Beauty: The Ugly Truth about Cosmetics." *American Nurse Today* 6, no. 5 (2011). Accessed March 5, 2012. https://www.americannursetoday.com/toxic-beauty-the-ugly-truth-about-cosmetics/.

[156] Ibid.

[157] Ibid.

[158] "The 'Dirty Dozen' Ingredients Investigated in the David Suzuki Foundation Survey of Chemicals in Cosmetics." davidsuzuki.org. Accessed March 6, 2012. http://www.davidsuzuki.org/issues/downloads/Dirty-dozen-backgrounder.pdf.

[159] Ibid.

[160] Smallbone, Kieran, et al. "The Role of Acidity in Solid Tumour Growth and Invasion." *Journal of Theoretical Biology* 235 (2005): 476–84.

[161] Robey, Ian F., et al. "Bicarbonate Increases Tumor pH and Inhibits Spontaneous Metastases." *Cancer Research* 69, no. 2260 (2009). Accessed March 14, 2012. http://cancerres.aacrjournals.org/content/69/6/2260.abstract.

[162] Rofstad, Einar K., et al. "Acidic Extracellular pH Promotes Experimental Metastasis of Human Melanoma Cells in Athymic Nude Mice." *Cancer Research* 66 (2006). Accessed March 5, 2012. http://cancerres.aacrjournals.org/content/66/13/6699.abstract?ijkey=6f1de3dcb24df43416f5003b8f892f1b6fd9d741&keytype2=tf_ipsecsha.

[163] Cover, C. M., et al. "Indole-3-Carbinol Inhibits the Expression of Cyclin-Dependent Kinase-6 and Induces a G1 Cell Cycle Arrest of Human Breast Cancer Cells Independent of Estrogen Receptor Signaling." *The Journal of Biological Chemistry* 273 (1998): 3838–47.

[164] Chen, I., et al. "Indole-3-Carbinol and Diindolylmethane as Aryl Hydrocarbon (Ah) Receptor Agonists and Antagonists in T47D Human Breast Cancer Cells." *Biochemical Pharmacology* 51 (1996): 1069–76.

[165] Verhagen H., et al. "Reduction of Oxidative DNA-Damage in Humans by Brussels Sprouts." *Carcinogenesis* 16 (1995): 969–70.

[166] Verhoeven D. T., et al. "Epidemiological Studies on Brassica Vegetables and Cancer Risk." *Cancer Epidemiology, Biomarkers and Prevention* 5, no. 9 (September 1996): 733–48.

[167] "Discovery May Help Scientists Boost Broccoli's Cancer-Fighting Power." EurekAlert! Accessed March 2, 2012.

[168] "Chlorophyll and Chlorophyllin." Linus Pauling Institute at Oregon State University. Accessed January 3, 2012. http://lpi.oregonstate.edu/infocenter/phytochemicals/chlorophylls/index.html#biological_activity.

[169] Cha, K. H., S. Y. Koo, and D. U. Lee. "Antiproliferative Effects of Carotenoids Extracted from *Chlorella ellipsoidea* and *Chlorella vulgaris* on Human Colon Cancer Cells." *Journal of Agricultural and Food Chemistry* 56, no. 22 (2008): 10521–26.

[170] Mathew, B., R. Sankaranarayanan, P. P. Nair, C. Varghese, T. Somanathan, B. P. Amma, et al. "Evaluation of Chemoprevention of Oral Cancer with *Spirulina fusiformis.*" *Nutrition and Cancer* 24, no. 2 (1995): 197–202.

[171] Maeda, N., et al. "Anti-Cancer Effect of Spinach Glycoglycerolipids as Angiogenesis Inhibitors Based on the Selective Inhibition of DNA Polymerase Activity." *Mini Reviews in Medicinal Chemistry* 11 (2011). Accessed March 3, 2012. http://www.ncbi.nlm.nih.gov/pubmed/21034405.

[172] Blot, W. J., J. Y. Li, P. R. Taylor, et al. "Nutrition Intervention Trials in Linxian, China: Supplementation with Specific Vitamin/Mineral Combinations, Cancer Incidence, and Disease-Specific Mortality in the General Population." *Journal of the National Cancer Institute* 85 (1993): 1483–91.

[173] Tanaka, T., M. Shminimizu, and H. Moriwaki. "Cancer Chemoprevention by Carotenoids." *Molecules* 17, no. 3 (March 14, 2012): 3202–42. Accessed March 27, 2012. http://www.ncbi.nlm.nih.gov/pubmed/22418926.

[174] Pinela, J., et al. "Nutritional Composition and Antioxidant Activity of Four Tomato (*Lycopersicon esculentum* L.) Farmers' Varieties in Northeastern Portugal Home Gardens." *Food and Chemical Toxicology* 50, no. 3–4 (2011): 829–34.

[175] "Fiber." University of Maryland Medical Center. Accessed December 3, 2012. http://www.umm.edu/altmed/articles/fiber-000303.htm.

[176] HealthDay. "High-Fiber Diet May Thwart Colon Cancer." USATODAY.com. Accessed March 28, 2012.

[177] "Uterine Cancer—2—Endometrial Cancer, Vitamin A, Vitamin C—Life Extension Health Concern." Life Extension. Accessed March 28, 2012.

[178] Owen, R. W., R. Haubner, G. Wurtele, E. Hull, B. Spiegelhalder, and H. Bartsch. "Olives and Olive Oil in Cancer Prevention." *European Journal of Cancer Prevention* 13, no. 4 (August 2004): 319–26.

[179] Menendez, J. A., and R. Lupu. "Mediterranean Dietary Traditions for the Molecular Treatment of Human Cancer: Anti-oncogenic Actions of the Main Olive Oil's Monounsaturated Fatty Acid Oleic Acid (18:1n-9)." *Current Pharmaceutical Biotechnology* 7, no. 6 (December 2006): 495–502.

[180] Menendez, Javier A., Alejandro Vazquez-Martin, Rocio Garcia-Villalba, Alegria Carrasco-Pancorbo, Cristina Oliveras-Ferraros, Alberto Fernandez-Gutierrez, and Antonio Segura-Carretero. "Anti-HER2 (erbB-2) Oncogene Effects of Phenolic Compounds Directly Isolated from Commercial Extra-Virgin Olive Oil (EVOO)." *BMC Cancer* 8 (December 18, 2008): 377.

[181] Choi, Hyun Ju, Do Young Lim, and Jung Han Yoon Park. "Induction of G1 and G2/M Cell Cycle Arrests by the Dietary Compound 3,3'-diindolylmethane in HT-29 Human Colon Cancer Cells." *BMC Gastroenterology* 9, no. 39 (2009).

[182] Bhatnagar, N. "3,3'-diindolylmethane Enhances the Efficacy of Butyrate in Colon Cancer Prevention through Down-Regulation of Survivin." *Cancer Prevention Research* 2, no. 6 (2009): 581–89.

[183] Schnäbele, K., et al. "Effects of Carrot and Tomato Juice Consumption on Faecal Markers Relevant to Colon Carcinogenesis in Humans." *The British Journal of Nutrition* 99, no. 3 (2008): 606–13. Accessed March 13, 2012. http://www.ncbi.nlm.nih.gov/pubmed/18254985.

[184] "Tea." Linus Pauling Institute at Oregon State University. Accessed January 3, 2012. http://lpi.oregonstate.edu/infocenter/phytochemicals/tea/.

[185] "Green Tea Extract Appears to Keep Cancer in Check in Majority of CLL Patients." Mayo Clinic. Accessed January 3, 2012.

[186] Okello, E. J., G. J. McDougall, S. Kumar, and C.J. Seal. "In Vitro Protective Effects of Colon-Available Extract of *Camellia sinensis* (Tea) against Hydrogen Peroxide and Beta-amyloid ($A\beta_{(1-42)}$) Induced Cytotoxicity in Differentiated PC12 Cells." *Phytomedicine* 18, no. 8–9 (June 15, 2011): 691–96. doi:10.1016/j.phymed.2010.11.004.

[187] Yeh, Jan-Ying, et al. "Antioxidant Properties and Antioxidant Compounds of Various Extracts from the Edible Basidiomycete *Grifola frondosa* (Maitake)." *Molecules* 16, no. 4 (2011): 3197–211.

[188] Chan, J. Y., et al. "Enhancement of In Vitro and In Vivo Anticancer Activities of Polysaccharide Peptide from *Grifola frondosa* by Chemical Modifications." *Pharmaceutical Biology* 49, no. 11 (2011): 1114–20.

[189] Masuda, Y. "A Polysaccharide Extracted from *Grifola frondosa* Enhances the Antitumor Activity of Bone Marrow-Derived Dendritic Cell-Based Immunotherapy against Murine Colon Cancer." *Cancer Immunology, Immunotherapy* 59, no. 10 (2009): 1531–41.

[190] Fullerton, S. A. "Induction of Apoptosis in Human Prostatic Cancer Cells with Beta-glucan (Maitake Mushroom Polysaccharide)." *Molecular Urology* 4, no. 1 (2000): 7–13.

[191] Tanaka, K., et al. "Oral Ingestion of *Lentinula edodes* Mycelia Extract Inhibits B16 Melanoma Growth via Mitigation of Regulatory T Cell-Mediated Immunosuppression." *Cancer Science* 102, no. 3 (2011): 516–21.

[192] Israilides, C., et al. "In Vitro Cytostatic and Immunomodulatory Properties of the Medicinal Mushrooms *Lentinula edodes*." *Phytomedicine* 15, no. 6–7 (June 2008): 512–19.

[193] Sliva, Daniel. "*Ganoderma lucidum* (Reishi) in Cancer Treatment." *Integrative Cancer Therapies* 2, no. 4 (2003): 358–64.

[194] Das, Shonkor Kumar, et al. "Medicinal Uses of the Mushroom *Cordyceps militaris*: Current State and Prospects." *Fitoterapia* 81, no. 8 (December 2010): 961–68.

[195] Chen, S., et al. "Anti-aromatase Activity of Phytochemicals in White Button Mushrooms." *Cancer Research* 66 (December 15, 2006):12026–34.

[196] Burtin, Patricia. "Nutritional Value of Seaweed." Electronic Journal of Environmental, Agricultural and Food Chemistry (2003). Accessed January 3, 2012.

[197] Ermakova, S., et al. "Fucoidans from Brown Seaweeds *Sargassum horneri*, *Eclonia cava*, *Costaria costata*: Structural Characteristics and Anticancer Activity." *Applied Biochemistry and Biotechnology* 164 (2011): 841.

[198] Gali-Muhtasib, H., M. Diab-Assaf, C. Boltze, J. Al-Hmaira, R. Hartig, et al. "Thymoquinone Extracted from Black Seed Triggers Apoptotic Cell Death in Human Colorectal Cancer Cells Via a p53-dependent Mechanism." *International Journal of Oncology* (October 2004).

[199] Salim, E. I., and S. Fukushima. "Chemopreventive Potential of Volatile Oil from Black Cumin (*Nigella sativa* L.) Seeds against Rat Colon Carcinogenesis." *Nutrition and Cancer* (2003).

[200] Duessel, S., et al. "Growth Inhibition of Human Colon Cancer Cells by Plant Compounds." *Clinical Laboratory Science* 21, no. 3 (Summer 2008): 151–57.

[201] Chan, M. M., C. T. Ho, and H. I. Huang. "Effects of Three Dietary Phytochemicals from Tea, Rosemary and Turmeric on Inflammation-Induced Nitrite Production." *Cancer Letters* 96 (1995): 23–29.

[202] Cheung, S., et al. "Anti-proliferative and Antioxidant Properties of Rosemary *Rosmarinus officinalis.*" *Oncology Reports* 17, no. 6 (June 2007): 1525–31.

[203] Ho, C. H., et al., eds. "Phytochemicals in Tea and Rosemary and Their Cancer-Preventive Properties." In *Food Phytochemicals for Cancer Prevention II,* edited by C. T. Ho, et al., 2–19. Washington, DC: American Chemical Society, 1994.

[204] "Pepper Component Hot Enough to Trigger Suicide in Prostate Cancer Cells." Cedars-Sinai Hospital. Accessed March 15, 2006.

[205] Johnson, J. J. "Carnosol: A Promising Anti-cancer and Anti-inflammatory Agent." *Cancer Letters* 305, no. 1 (2011): 1–7. Accessed March 12, 2012. http://www.ncbi.nlm.nih.gov/pubmed/21382660.

[206] "Parsley, Celery Carry Crucial Component for Fight against Breast Cancer, Study Suggests." Science Daily. Accessed March 21, 2012. http://www.sciencedaily.com/releases/2011/05/110509122732.htm.

[207] Roberts, L. J., M. G. Traber, and B. Frei. "Vitamins E and C in the Prevention of Cardiovascular Disease and Cancer in Men." *Free Radical Biology and Medicine* 46, no. 11 (2009): 1558.

[208] Zhang S., D. J. Hunter, M. R. Forman, et al. "Dietary Carotenoids and Vitamins A, C, and E and Risk of Breast Cancer." *Journal of the National Cancer Institute* 91, no. 6 (1999): 547–56.

[209] Feiz, H. R., and S. Mobarhan. "Does Vitamin C Intake Slow the Progression of Gastric Cancer in *Helicobacter pylori*-Infected Populations?" *Nutrition Reviews* 60, no. 1 (2002): 34–36.

[210] Chen, Q., M. G. Espey, A. Y. Sun, et al. "Pharmacologic Doses of Ascorbate Act as a Prooxidant and Decrease Growth of Aggressive Tumor Xenografts in Mice." *Proceedings of the National Academy of Sciences* 105, no. 32 (2008): 11105–9.

[211] Drisko, J. A., J. Chapman, and V. J. Hunter. "The Use of Antioxidants with First-Line Chemotherapy in Two Cases of Ovarian Cancer." *Journal of the American College of Nutrition* 22, no. 2 (2003):118–23.

[212] Gonzalez, Michael, et al. "Orthomolecular Oncology Review: Ascorbic Acid and Cancer 25 Years Later." *Integrated Cancer Therapies* 4 (March 2005): 32–44.

[213] Moss, Ralph. "Should Patients Undergoing Chemotherapy and Radiotherapy Be Prescribed Antioxidants?" *Integrative Cancer Therapies.* Accessed March 28, 2012. http://ict.sagepub.com/content/5/1/63.abstract.

[214] van de Mark, K., et al. "Alpha-lipoic Acid Induces p27Kip-Dependent Cell Cycle Arrest in Non-transformed Cell Lines and Apoptosis in Tumor Cell Lines." *Journal of Cellular Physiology* 194, no. 3 (2003): 325–40.

[215] Lee, H. S., et al. "Alpha-Lipoic Acid Reduces Matrix Metalloproteinase Activity in MDA-MB-231 Human Breast Cancer Cells." *Nutrition Research* 30, no. 6 (June 2010): 403–9.

216 Myzak, M. C., and A. C. Carr. "Myeloperoxidase-Dependent Caspase-3 Activation and Apoptosis in HL-60 Cells: Protection by the Antioxidants Ascorbate and (Dihydro) lipoic Acid." *Redox Report* 7, no. 1 (2002): 47–53. Accessed March 13, 2012. http://www.ncbi.nlm.nih.gov/pubmed/11981455.

217 Brown, M. D. "Promotion of Prostatic Metastatic Migration towards Human Bone Marrow Stoma by Omega 6 and Its Inhibition by Omega 3 PUFAs." *British Journal of Cancer* 94, no. 6 (2006): 842–53.

218 Gago-Dominguez, M. "Opposing Effects of Dietary n-3 and n-6 Fatty Acids on Mammary Carcinogenesis: The Singapore Chinese Health Study." *British Journal of Cancer* 89, no. 9 (2003): 1686–92.

219 MacLean, C., et al. "Effects of Omega-3 Fatty Acids on Cancer." *AHRQ Evidence Reports* (February 2005).

220 Prakash, P., N. I. Krinsky, and R. M. Russell. "Retinoids, Carotenoids, and Human Breast Cancer Cell Cultures: A Review of Differential Effects." *Nutrition Reviews* 58, no. 6 (2000): 170–76.

221 "Vitamin A May Slash Melanoma Risk, Especially in Women." LiveScience. Accessed March 28, 2012.

222 de Klerk, N. H., A. W. Musk, G. L. Ambrosini, et al. "Vitamin A and Cancer Prevention II: Comparison of the Effects of Retinol and Beta-carotene." *International Journal of Cancer* 75 (1998): 362–67.

223 Sivakumaran, Muttuswamy. "Role of Vitamin A Deficiency in the Pathogenesis of Myeloproliferative Disorders." *Blood Journal* 98 (2001): 1636–37. Accessed March 28, 2012. http://bloodjournal.hematologylibrary.org/content/98/5/1636.full.

224 Li, K., et al. "The Effect of Vitamin A Deficiency in Maternal Rats on Tumor Formation in Filial Rats." *Journal of Pediatric Surgery* 44, no. 3 (2009): 565–70. Accessed March 12, 2012. http://www.ncbi.nlm.nih.gov/pubmed/19302860.

225 Ruano-Ravina, A., A. Figueiras, and J. M. Barros-Dios. "Diet and Lung Cancer: A New Approach." *European Journal of Cancer Prevention* 9 (2000): 395–400.

226 DiGiovanna, J. J. "Retinoid Chemoprevention in Patients at High Risk for Skin Cancer." *Medical and Pediatric Oncology* 36 (2001): 564–67.

227 Null, Gary. *The Complete Encyclopedia of Natural Healing.* New York: Kensington, 1998.

228 Gallicchio, L., K. Boyd, G. Matanoski, et al. "Carotenoids and the Risk of Developing Lung Cancer: A Systematic Review." *American Journal of Clinical Nutrition* 88, no. 2 (August 2008): 372–83.

229 Yang, T., X. Yang, X. Wang, Y. Wang, Z. Song. "The Role of Tomato Products and Lycopene in the Prevention of Gastric Cancer: A Meta-analysis of Epidemiologic Studies." *Medical Hypotheses* 80, no. 4 (April 2013): 383–88.

230 Etminan, M., B. Takkouche, F. Caamano-Isorna. "The Role of Tomato Products and Lycopene in the Prevention of Prostate Cancer: A Meta-analysis of Observational Studies." *Cancer Epidemiology Biomarkers and Prevention* 13, no. 3 (2004): 340–45.

231 Cui, Y., J. M. Shikany, S. Liu, et al. "Selected Antioxidants and Risk of Hormone Receptor-Defined Invasive Breast Cancers among Postmenopausal Women in the Women's Health Initiative Observational Study." *American Journal of Clinical Nutrition* 87, no. 4 (April 2008): 1009–18.

[232] Cho, E., et al. "Premenopausal Intakes of Vitamins A, C, and E, Folate, and Carotenoids, and Risk of Breast Cancer." *Cancer Epidemiology, Biomarkers and Prevention* 12, no. 8 (August 2003): 713–20.

[233] Zhang, Shumin, et al. "Dietary Carotenoids and Vitamins A, C, and E and Risk of Breast Cancer." *Journal of the National Cancer Institute* 91, no. 6 (March 17, 1999): 547–56.

[234] Knekt, Paul. "Dietary Flavonoids and the Risk of Lung Cancer and Other Malignant Neoplasms." *American Journal of Epidemiology* 146, no. 3 (August 1, 1997): 223–30.

[235] Le Marchand, Loïc, et al. "Intake of Flavonoids and Lung Cancer." *Journal of the National Cancer Institute* 91, no. 2 (January 19, 2000): 154–60.

[236] Cui, Y., et al. "Dietary Flavonoid Intake and Lung Cancer—A Population-Based Case-Control Study." *Cancer* 112, no. 10 (May 15, 2008): 2241–48.

[237] "Vitamin E." Linus Pauling Institute at Oregon State University. Accessed March 21, 2012. http://lpi.oregonstate.edu/infocenter/vitamins/vitaminE/.

[238] "Vitamin E in Front Line of Prostate Cancer Fight." Science Daily. Accessed March 8, 2012. http://www.sciencedaily.com/releases/2010/10/101019111718.htm.

[239] Null, *Encyclopedia of Natural Healing.*

[240] Li, L., et al. "Induction of Apoptosis in Hepatocellular Carcinoma Smmc-7721 Cells by Vitamin K(2) Is Associated with p53 and Independent of the Intrinsic Apoptotic Pathway." *Molecular and Cellular Biochemistry* 342, no. 1–2 (September 2010): 125–31.

[241] Nimptsch, Katharina. "Dietary Vitamin K Intake in Relation to Cancer Incidence and Mortality: Results from the Heidelberg Cohort of the European Prospective Investigation into Cancer and Nutrition." *American Journal of Clinical Nutrition* 10 (2010): 3945. Accessed March 13, 2012. http://www.ajcn.org/content/early/2010/03/24/ajcn.2009.28691.abstract.

[242] Kaneda, M., D. Zhang, R. Bhattacharjee, K. Nakahama, S. Arii, and I. Morita. "Vitamin K2 Suppresses Malignancy of HuH7 Hepatoma Cells via Inhibition of Connexin 43." *Cancer Letters* 263 (2008): 53–60.

[243] Amaral, Andre, et al. "Selenium and Bladder Cancer Risk: A Meta-analysis." *Cancer Epidemiology, Biomarkers and Prevention* (August 2010).

[244] Duffield-Lillico, A. J., et al. "Selenium Supplementation, Baseline Plasma Selenium Status and Incidence of Prostate Cancer: An Analysis of the Complete Treatment Period of the Nutritional Prevention of Cancer Trial." *BJU International* 91, no. 7 (2003): 608–12.

[245] Bleys, J., et al. "Serum Selenium Levels and All-Cause, Cancer, and Cardiovascular Mortality among U.S. Adults." *Archives of Internal Medicine* 168, no. 4 (2008): 404–10.

[246] Syed, Deeba, et al. "Chemoprevention of Prostate Cancer through Dietary Agents: Progress and Promise." *Cancer Epidemiology, Biomarkers and Prevention* 16, no. 11 (November 2007): 2193–203.

[247] Lah, J. J., W. Cui, and K. Q. Hu. "Effects and Mechanisms of Silibinin on Human Hepatoma Cell Lines." *World Journal of Gastroenterology* 13, no. 40 (2007): 5299–305.

[248] Kiefer, Dale. "Report: A New Weapon to Fight Prostate Cancer." *Life Extension Magazine* (November 2005). Accessed March 3, 2012. http://www.lef.org/magazine/mag2005/nov2005_report_prostate_01.htm.

[249] Null, *Encyclopedia of Natural Healing.*

[250] Sakano, K., et al. "Suppression of Azoxymethane-Induced Colonic Premalignant Lesion Formation by Coenzyme Q10 in Rats." *Asian Pacific Journal of Cancer Prevention* 7, no. 4 (October–December 2006): 599–603.

[251] Rusciani, L., et al. "Recombinant Interferon Alpha-2b and Coenzyme Q10 as a Post-surgical Adjuvant Therapy for Melanoma: A 3-Year Trial with Recombinant Interferon-Alpha and 5-Year Follow-Up." *Melanoma Research* 17, no. 3 (June 2007): 177–83.

[252] Folklers, K., et al. "Activities of Vitamin Q10 in Animal Models and a Serious Deficiency in Patients with Cancer." *Biochemical and Biophysical Research Communications* 234, no. 2 (May 19, 1997): 296–99.

[253] Kaur, Manjinder, et al. "Anticancer and Cancer Chemopreventive Potential of Grape Seed Extract and Other Grape-Based Products." *Journal of Nutrition* 139, no. 9 (September 2009): 1806S–12S.

[254] Radhakrishnan, S. "Resveratrol Potentiates Grape Seed Extract Induced Human Colon Cancer Cell Apoptosis." *Frontiers in Bioscience* 3 (June 1, 2011): 1509–23.

[255] Raina, Komal, et al. "Oral Grape Seed Extract Inhibits Prostate Tumor Growth and Progression in TRAMP Mice." *Cancer Research* 67, no. 12 (June 15, 2007): 5976–82.

[256] Chen, Changjie, et al. "Grape Seed Extract Inhibits Proliferation of Breast Cancer Cell MCF-7 and Decreases the Gene Expression of Survivin." *China Journal of Chinese Materia Medica* 34, no. 4 (February 2009): 433–37.

[257] Null, *Encyclopedia of Natural Healing.*

[258] Wise, D., and C. Thompson. "Glutamine Addiction: A New Therapeutic Target in Cancer." *Trends in Biochemical Sciences* 35, no. 8 (August 2010): 427–33.

[259] Villareal, D. T., and J. O. Holloszy. "Effect of DHEA on Abdominal Fat and Insulin Action in Elderly Women and Men: A Randomized Controlled Trial." *JAMA* 292, no. 18 (2004); 2243–48.

[260] Smith, Timothy J. *Renewal: The Anti-Aging Revolution.* Rodale Press, 1998.

[261] Jung, Brittney, and Nihal Ahmad. "Melatonin in Cancer Management: Progress and Promise." *Cancer Research* 66, no. 20 (October 15, 2006): 9789–93.

[262] Megdal, S. P., et al. "Night Work and Breast Cancer Risk: A Systematic Review and Meta-analysis." *European Journal of Cancer* 41, no. 13 (September 2005): 2023–32.

[263] Lissoni, P., S. Barni, A. Ardizzoia, G. Tancini, A. Conti, and G. Maestroni. "A Randomized Study with the Pineal Hormone Melatonin Versus Supportive Care Alone in Patients with Brain Metastases Due to Solid Neoplasms." *Cancer* 73, no. 3 (February 1, 1994): 699–701.

[264] Schernhammer, Eva, and Susan E. Hankinson. "Urinary Melatonin Levels and Post-menopausal Breast Cancer Risk in the Nurses' Health Study Cohort." *Cancer Epidemiology, Biomarkers and Prevention* 18, no. 1 (January 2009): 74–79.

[265] Park, S. Y., et al. "Melatonin Suppresses Tumor Angiogenesis by Inhibiting HIF-1alpha Stabilization Under Hypoxia." *Journal of Pineal Research* 48, no. 2 (March 2010): 178–84.

[266] Beuth, J. "Proteolytic Enzyme Therapy in Evidence-Based Complementary Oncology: Fact or Fiction?" *Integrative Cancer Therapies* 7, no. 4 (December 2008).

[267] Yamashita, Keishi, et al. "A Tumor-Suppressive Role for Trypsin in Human Cancer Progression." *Cancer Research* 63 (2003). Accessed March 5, 2012. http://cancerres. aacrjournals.org/content/63/20/6575.full.

[268] Wald, M., et al. "Mixture of Trypsin, Chymotrypsin and Papain Reduces Formation of Metasteses and Extends Survival Time of C57B16 Mice with Syngeneic Melanoma B16." *Cancer Chemotherapy and Pharmacology* 47 (July 2001): S16–22.

[269] Larsson, S. C., et al. "High-Fat Dairy Food and Conjugated Linoleic Acid Intakes in Relation to Colorectal Cancer." *American Journal of Clinical Nutrition* 82, no. 4 (October 2005): 894–900.

[270] Chen, B. Q., et al. "Inhibitory Effects of c9, t11-Conjugated Linoleic Acid." *World Journal of Gastroenterology* 9, no. 9 (September 2003): 1909–14.

[271] Aro, A., et al. "Inverse Association Between Dietary and Serum." *Nutrition and Cancer* 38, no. 2 (2000): 151–57.

[272] Ip, C., J. A. Scimeca, and H. J. Thompson. "Conjugated Linoleic Acid: A Powerful Anticarcinogen from Animal Fat Sources." *Cancer* 74, no. 3 (August 1994): 1050–54.

[273] Kritchevsky, D. "Antimutagenic and Some Other Effects of Conjugated Linoleic Acid." *The British Journal of Nutrition* 83, no. 5 (May 2000): 459–65.

[274] Bhattacharya, A., J. Banu, M. Rahman, J. Causey, and G. Fernandes. "Biological Effects of Conjugated Linoleic Acids in Health and Disease." *Journal of Nutritional Biochemistry* 17, no. 12 (December 2006): 789–810.

[275] Johnson K. D., O. V. Glinskii, V. V. Mossine, et al. "Galectin-3 as a Potential Therapeutic Target in Tumors Arising from Malignant Endothelia." *Neoplasia* 9, no. 8 (August 2007): 662–70.

[276] Gupta G. P., and J. Massague. "Cancer Metastasis: Building a Framework." *Cell* 127, no. 4 (November 17, 2006): 679–95.

[277] Strum, S., M. Scholz, J. McDermed, M. McCulloch, I. Eliaz. "Modified Citrus Pectin Slows PSA Doubling Time: A Pilot Clinical Trial." Paper presented at the International Conference on Diet and Prevention of Cancer, Tampere, Finland, May 1999.

[278] Guess B. W., M. C. Scholz, S. B. Strum, et al. "Modified Citrus Pectin (MCP) Increases the Prostate-Specific Antigen Doubling Time in Men with Prostate Cancer: A Phase II Pilot Study." *Prostate Cancer and Prostatic Diseases* 6, no. 4 (2003): 301–4.

[279] Ushida, Y., K. Sekine, T. Kuhara, N. Takasuka, M. Iigo, and H. Tsuda. "Inhibitory Effects of Bovine Lactoferrin on Intestinal Polyposis in the Apc(Min) Mouse." *Cancer Letters* 134, no. 2 (December 25, 1998): 141–45.

[280] Yoo, Y. C., S. Watanabe, R. Watanabe, K. Hata, K. Shimazaki, and I. Azuma. "Bovine Lactoferrin and Lactoferricin, a Peptide Derived from Bovine Lactoferrin, Inhibit Tumor Metastasis in Mice." *Japanese Journal of Cancer Research* 88, no. 2 (February 1997): 184–90.

[281] Sakamoto, N. "Antitumor Effect of Human Lactoferrin against Newly Established Human Pancreatic Cancer Cell Line SPA." *Gan to Kagaku Ryoho* 25, no. 10 (August 1998): 1557–63.

[282] Tsuda, H., K. Sekine, J. Nakamura, Y. Ushida, T. Kuhara, N. Takasuka, et al. "Inhibition of Azoxymethane Initiated Colon Tumor and Aberrant Crypt Foci Development

by Bovine Lactoferrin Administration in F344 Rats." *Advances in Experimental Medicine and Biology* 443 (1998): 273–84.

[283] Li, J., H. J. Tu, G. Dai, et al. "N-acetyl Cysteine Inhibits Human Signet Ring Cell Gastric Cancer Cell Line (SJ-89) Cell Growth by Inducing Apoptosis and DNA Synthesis Arrest." *European Journal of Gastroenterology and Hepatology* 19, no. 9 (September 2007): 769–74.

[284] Yang, J., Y. Su, and A. Richmond. "Antioxidants Tiron and N-acetyl-L-cysteine Differentially Mediate Apoptosis in Melanoma Cells via a Reactive Oxygen Species-Independent NF-kappaB Pathway." *Free Radical Biology and Medicine* 42, no. 9 (May 2007): 1369–80.

[285] Balansky, R., G. Ganchev, M. Iltcheva, V. E. Steele, and S. De Flora. "Prevention of Cigarette Smoke-Induced Lung Tumors in Mice by Budesonide, Phenethyl Isothiocyanate, and N-acetyl Cysteine." *International Journal of Cancer* 126, no. 5 (March 1, 2010): 1047–54.

[286] Guan, D., Y. Xu, M. Yang, H. Wang, X. Wang, and Z. Shen. "N-acetyl Cysteine and Penicillamine Induce Apoptosis via the ER Stress Response-Signaling Pathway." *Molecular Carcinogenesis* 49, no. 1 (January 2010): 68–74.

[287] Fares, R., et al. "The Antioxidant and Anti-proliferative Activity of the Lebanese *Olea europaea* Extract." *Plant Foods in Human Nutrition* 66, no. 1 (March 2011): 58–63.

[288] Bouallagui, Z., et al. "Hydroxytyrosol Rich Extract from Olive Leaves Modulates Cell Cycle Progression in Mcf-7 Human Breast Cancer Cells." *Food and Chemical Toxicology* 49, no. 1 (January 2011): 179–84.

[289] Mijatovic, S., et al. "Multiple Antimelanoma Potential of Dry Olive Leaf Extract." *International Journal of Cancer* 128, no. 8 (April 15, 2011): 1955–65.

[290] Arthur, G., and R. Bittman. "The Inhibition of Cell Signaling Pathways by Antitumor Ether Lipids." *Biochimica et Biophysica Acta* 1390, no. 1 (February 5, 1998): 85–102.

[291] Samadder, P., C. Richards, R. Bittman, R. P. Bhullar, and G. Arthur. "The Antitumor Ether Lipid 1-Q-octadecyl-2-O-methyl-rac-glycerophosphocholine (ET-18-OCH3) Inhibits the Association between Ras and Raf-1." *Anticancer Research* 23, no. 3B (May 2003): 2291–95.

[292] Pedrono, F., N. A. Khan, A. B. Legrand. "Regulation of Calcium Signalling by 1-O-alkylglycerols in Human Jurkat T Lymphocytes." *Life Sciences* 74, no. 22 (April 16, 2004): 2793–801.

[293] Brohult A., and J. Holmberg. "Alkoxyglycerols in the Treatment of Leukopaenia Caused by Irradiation." *Nature* 174, no. 4441 (December 11, 1954): 1102–3.

[294] Jang, M., L. Cai, G. O. Udeani, et al. "Cancer Chemopreventive Activity of Resveratrol, a Natural Product Derived from Grapes." *Science* 275, no. 5297 (1997): 218–20.

[295] Fulda, S., and K. M. Debatin. "Resveratrol Modulation of Signal Transduction in Apoptosis and Cell Survival: A Mini-Review." *Cancer Detection and Prevention* 30, no. 3 (2006): 217–23.

[296] Woo, J. H., J. H. Lim, Y. H. Kim, et al. "Resveratrol Inhibits Phorbol Myristate Acetate-Induced Matrix Metalloproteinase-9 Expression by Inhibiting JNK and PKC Delta Signal Transduction." *Oncogene* 23, no. 10 (2004): 1845–53.

[297] Ciolino, H. P., and G. C. Yeh. "Inhibition of Aryl Hydrocarbon-Induced Cytochrome P-450 1A1 Enzyme Activity and CYP1A1 Expression by Resveratrol." *Molecular Pharmacology* 56, no. 4 (1999): 760–67.

[298] Joe, A. K., H. Liu, M. Suzui, M. E. Vural, D. Xiao, and I. B. Weinstein. "Resveratrol Induces Growth Inhibition, S-phase Arrest, Apoptosis, and Changes in Biomarker Expression in Several Human Cancer Cell Lines." *Clinical Cancer Research* 8, no. 3 (2002): 893–903.

[299] "Cancer Research—Bindweed." The Riordan Clinic Health Center in Wichita, KS. Accessed March 21, 2012.

[300] Riordan, N. H., X. Meng, and H. D. Riordan. "Effects of Cell Wall Extracts of Gram Positive Bacteria (MPGC) on Human Immunity and Tumor Growth in Animals." Presentation at Comprehensive Cancer Care 2000, Arlington, Virginia, June 2000.

[301] Prasad, A. S., et al. "Dietary Zinc and Prostate Cancer in the TRAMP Mouse Model." *Journal of Medicinal Food* 13, no. 1 (February 2010): 70–76.

[302] Epstein, M. M., et al. "Dietary Zinc and Prostate Cancer Survival in a Swedish Cohort." *American Journal of Clinical Nutrition* 93, no. 3 (March 2011): 586–93.

[303] Song, W. O., O. K. Chun, I. Hwang, et al. "Soy Isoflavones as Safe Functional Ingredients." *Journal of Medicinal Food* 10, no. 4 (December 2007): 571–80.

[304] "Soy Compound May Halt Spread of Prostate Cancer." Science Daily. Accessed March 29, 2012. http://www.sciencedaily.com/releases/2008/03/080314085038.htm.

[305] Aboutalebi, S., et al. "Immune Protection, Natural Products, and Skin Cancer: Is There Anything New under the Sun?" *Journal of Drugs in Dermatology* 5, no. 6 (June 2006): 512–17.

[306] Pecere, Teresa, et al. "Aloe-emodin Is a New Type of Anticancer Agent with Selective Activity against Neuroectodermal Tumors." *Cancer Research* 60 (2000). Accessed March 14, 2012. http://cancerres.aacrjournals.org/content/60/11/2800.short.

[307] Corsi, M. M., et al. "The Therapeutic Potential of Aloe Vera in Tumor-Bearing Rats." *International Journal of Tissue Reactions* 20, no. 4 (1998): 115–18. Accessed March 12, 2012. http://ukpmc.ac.uk/abstract/MED/10093794/reload=0;jsessionid=tdlDotXQ VWctw7ukpVz9.2.

[308] Duan, P., and Z. Wang. "Clinical Study on Effect of Astragalus in Efficacy Enhancing and Toxicity Reducing of Chemotherapy in Patients of Malignant Tumor." *Zhongguo Zhong Xi Yi Jie He Za Zhi* 22, no. 7 (July 2002): 515–17.

[309] Cui, R., J. He, B. Wang, et al. "Suppressive Effect of Astragalus Membranaceus Bunge on Chemical Hepatocarcinogenesis in Rats." *Cancer Chemotherapy and Pharmacology* 51, no. 1 (January 2003): 75–80.

[310] Cho, W. C., and K. N. Leung. "In Vitro and In Vivo Anti-tumor Effects of Astragalus Membranaceus." *Cancer Letters* 252, no. 1 (July 8, 2007): 43–54.

[311] Auyeung, K. K., P. K. Woo, P. C. Law, and J. K. Ko. "Astragalus Saponins Modulate Cell Invasiveness and Angiogenesis in Human Gastric Adenocarcinoma Cells." *Journal of Ethnopharmacology* 141, no. 2 (June 2012): 635–41.

[312] Pretner, E., H. Amri, W. Li, et al. "Cancer-Related Overexpression of the Peripheral-Type Benzodiazepine Receptor and Cytostatic Anticancer Effects of Ginkgo Biloba Extract (EGb 761)." *Anticancer Research* 26, no. 1A (2006): 9–22.

313 Xu, A. H., H. S. Chen, B. C. Sun, X. R. Xiang, Y. F. Chu, F. Zhai, and L. C. Jia. "Therapeutic Mechanism of Ginkgo Biloba Exocarp Polysaccharides on Gastric Cancer." *World Journal of Gastroenterology* 9, no. 11 (2003): 2424–27.

314 Ye, B., M. Aponte, Y. Dai, et al. "Ginkgo Biloba and Ovarian Cancer Prevention: Epidemiological and Biological Evidence." *Cancer Letters* 251, no. 1 (2007): 43–52.

315 Block, Keith, and Mark Mead. "Immune System Effects of Echinacea, Ginseng, and Astragalus: A Review." *Integrative Cancer Therapies* 3 (2003). Accessed March 6, 2012. http://www.comilac.com.tr/uploads/pdf/galuskaynak2.pdf.

316 Fleischauer, A., et al. "Garlic Consumption and Cancer Prevention: Meta-analyses of Colorectal and Stomach Cancers." *American Journal of Clinical Nutrition* 72, no. 4 (October 2000): 1047–52.

317 Nqo, S., et al. "Does Garlic Reduce Risk of Colorectal Cancer? A Systematic Review." *Journal of Nutrition* 137, no. 10 (October 2007): 2264–69.

318 Hong, Y. S., et al. "Effects of Allyl Sulfur Compounds and Garlic Extract on the Expression of Bcl-2, Bax, and p53 in Non Small Cell Lung Cancer Cell Lines." *Experimental and Molecular Medicine* 32, no. 3 (September 2000): 127–34.

319 Bhatia, Kanchan, et al. "Protective Effect of S-allylcysteine against Cyclophosphamide-Induced Bladder Hemorrhagic Cystitis in Mice." *Food and Chemical Toxicology* 46, no. 11 (2008). Accessed March 8, 2012. http://www.sciencedirect.com/science/article/pii/S0278691508004274.

320 "Dietary Ginger May Work Against Cancer Growth." Science Daily. Accessed March 29, 2012. http://www.sciencedaily.com/releases/2003/10/031029064357.htm.

321 Jeong, C. H., A. M. Bode, A. Pugliese, et al. "[6]-Gingerol Suppresses Colon Cancer Growth by Targeting Leukotriene A4 Hydrolase." *Cancer Research* 69, no. 13 (July 1, 2009): 5584–91.

322 Liu, R., et. al. "Expression and Function of Intracellular Fatty Acid-Binding Proteins in Human Malignant Glioma Cells and Tissues." Presentation at the 97th Annual Meeting of the American Association for Cancer Research, Washington, DC, 2006.

323 Borger, J. Everett. "How Curcumin Protects against Cancer." *Life Extension Magazine*. March 2011. Accessed March 9, 2012.

324 Ravindran, J., S. Prasad, and B. B. Aggarwal. "Curcumin and Cancer Cells: How Many Ways Can Curry Kill Tumor Cells Selectively?" *AAPS Journal* 11, no. 3 (September 2009): 495–510.

325 Zhang, J., Y. Du, C. Wu, et al. "Curcumin Promotes Apoptosis in Human Lung Adenocarcinoma Cells through miR-186* Signaling Pathway." *Oncology Reports* 24, no. 5 (November 2010): 1217–23.

326 Zhang, J., T. Zhang, X. Ti, et al. "Curcumin Promotes Apoptosis in A549/DDP Multidrug-Resistant Human Lung Adenocarcinoma Cells through an miRNA Signaling Pathway." *Biochemical and Biophysical Research Communications* 399, no. 1 (August 13, 2010): 1–6.

327 Clark, C. A., M. D. McEachern, S. H. Shah, et al. "Curcumin Inhibits Carcinogen and Nicotine-Induced Mammalian Target of Rapamycin Pathway Activation in Head and Neck Squamous Cell Carcinoma." *Cancer Prevention Research (Phila)* 3 no. 12 (December 2010): 1586–95.

328 Quiroga, A., P. L. Quiroga, E. Martinez, E. A. Soria, and M. A. Valentich. "Anti-breast Cancer Activity of Curcumin on the Human Oxidation-Resistant Cells ZR-75-1 with Gamma-glutamyl transpeptidase Inhibition." *Journal of Experimental Therapeutics and Oncology* 8, no. 3 (2010): 261–66.

329 Ibrahim, A., A. El-Meligy, H. Fetaih, A. Dessouki, G. Stoica, and R. Barhoumi. "Effect of Curcumin and Meriva on the Lung Metastasis of Murine Mammary Gland Adenocarcinoma." *In Vivo* 24, no. 4 (July–August 2010): 401–8.

330 Han, Y., T. Haraguchi, S. Iwanaga, et al. "Consumption of Some Polyphenols Reduces Fecal Deoxycholic Acid and Lithocholic Acid, the Secondary Bile Acids of Risk Factors of Colon Cancer." *Journal of Agricultural and Food Chemistry* 57, no. 18 (September 23, 2009): 8587–90.

331 Kang, J. H., K. H. Song, J. K. Woo, et al. "Ginsenoside Rp1 from Panax Ginseng Exhibits Anti-cancer Activity by Down-Regulation of the IGF-1R/Akt Pathway in Breast Cancer Cells." *Plant Foods for Human Nutrition* 66, no. 3 (September 2011): 298–305.

332 He, B. C., J. L. Gao, X. Luo, et al. "Ginsenoside Rg3 Inhibits Colorectal Tumor Growth through the Down-Regulation of Wnt/ß-catenin Signaling." *International Journal of Oncology* 38, no. 2 (February 2011): 437–45.

333 Yan, Amy. "University of California: Hot Tea or Hot Air? Immunomodulatory Effects of Panax Ginseng in the Prevention of Cancer." *Nutrition Bytes* 4, no. 1 (1998).

334 Sugiyama, Tomomi, and Yasuyuki Sadzuka. "Combination of Theanine with Doxorubicin Inhibits Hepatic Metastasis of M5076 Ovarian Sarcoma." *Clinical Cancer Research* 5, no. 2 (February 1999): 413–16.

335 Zhang, G., Y. Miura, and K. Yagasaki. "Effects of Dietary Powdered Green Tea and L-theanine on Tumor Growth and Endogenous Hyperlipidemia in Hepatoma-Bearing Rats." *Bioscience, Biotechnology, and Biochemistry* 66, no. 4 (2002): 711–16.

336 Sadzuka, Y., et al. "Improvement of Idarubicin Induced Antitumor Activity and Bone Marrow Suppression by Theanine, a Component of Tea." *Cancer Letters* 158, no. 2 (October 2000): 119–24.

337 Israilides, C., D. Kletsas, D. Arapoglou, et al. "In Vitro Cytostatic and Immunomodulatory Properties of the Medicinal Mushroom *Lentinula edodes*." *Phytomedicine* 15, no. 6 (June 2008): 512–9.

338 Ng, M. L., and A. T. Yap. "Inhibition of Human Colon Carcinoma Development by Lentinan from Shiitake Mushrooms (*Lentinus edodes*)." *Journal of Alternative and Complementary Medicine* 8, no. 5 (2002): 581–89.

339 Isoda, N., Y. Eguchi, H. Nukaya, et al. "Clinical Efficacy of Superfine Dispersed Lentinan (Beta-1,3-glucan) in Patients with Hepatocellular Carcinoma." *Hepatogastroenterology* 56, no. 90 (March–April 2009): 437–41.

340 Oba, K., M. Kobayashi, T. Matsui, Y. Kodera, and J. Sakamoto. "Individual Patient Based Meta-analysis of Lentinan for Unresectable/Recurrent Gastric Cancer." *Anticancer Research* 29, no. 7 (July 2009): 2739–45.

341 Shimizu, K., S. Watanabe, S. Watanabe, et al. "Efficacy of Oral Administered Superfine Dispersed Lentinan for Advanced Pancreatic Cancer." *Hepato-gastroenterology* 56, no. 89 (February 2009): 240–44.

342 Jantova, S., L. Cipak, and S. Letasiova. "Berberine Induces Apoptosis through a Mitochondrial/Caspase Pathway in Human Promonocytic U937 Cells." *Toxicol In Vitro* 21, no. 1 (February 2007): 25–31.

343 Serafim, T. L., P. J. Oliveira, V. A. Sardao, E. Perkins, D. Parke, and J. Holy. "Different Concentrations of Berberine Result in Distinct Cellular Localization Patterns and Cell Cycle Effects in a Melanoma Cell Line." *Cancer Chemotherapy and Pharmacology* 61, no. 6 (May 2008): 1007–18.

344 Mantena, S. K., S. D. Sharma, and S. K. Katiyar. "Berberine, a Natural Product, Induces G1-Phase Cell Cycle Arrest and Caspase-3-Dependent Apoptosis in Human Prostate Carcinoma Cells." *Molecular Cancer Therapeutics* 5, no. 2 (February 2006): 296–308.

345 Parada-Turska, J., R. Paduch, M. Majdan, M. Kandefer-Szerszen, and W. Rzeski. "Antiproliferative Activity of Parthenolide against Three Human Cancer Cell Lines and Human Umbilical Vein Endothelial Cells." *Pharmacological Reports* 59, no. 2 (March–April 2007): 233–37.

346 Curry, E. A., D. J. Murry, C. Yoder, et al. "Phase I Dose Escalation Trial of Feverfew with Standardized Doses of Parthenolide in Patients with Cancer." *Investigational New Drugs* 22, no. 3 (August 2004): 299–305.

347 Zhang, S., C. N. Ong, and H. M. Shen. "Involvement of Proapoptotic Bcl-2 Family Members in Parthenolide-Induced Mitochondrial Dysfunction and Apoptosis." *Cancer Letters* 211, no. 2 (August 10, 2004): 175–88.

348 Gerson Institute. "Dr. Max Gerson." Accessed September 16, 2013. http://gerson. org/gerpress/dr-max-gerson/.

349 Null, Gary. *Get Healthy Now! A Complete Guide to Prevention, Treatment, and Healthy Living.* New York: Seven Stories Press, 1999.

350 Ibid.

351 Ibid.

352 Ibid.

353 Null, *Get Healthy Now!*

354 Sodi-Pallares et al. "A Low Sodium, High Water, High Potassium Regimen in the Successful Management of Some Cardiovascular Diseases: Preliminary Clinical Report." *Canadian Medical Association Journal* 83, no. 6 (August 6, 1960).

355 Null, *Get Healthy Now!*

356 Null, *Get Healthy Now!*

357 Ibid.

358 Dr. Stanley Beyerle, interview by Gary Null, February 23, 1995.

359 McCarthy, Edward F. "The Toxins of William B. Coley and the Treatment of Bone and Soft-Tissue Sarcomas." *The Iowa Orthopaedic Journal* 26 (2006): 154–58.